Preparticipation Physical Evaluation

SECOND EDITION

Preparticipation Physical Evaluation

SECOND EDITION

American Academy of Family Physicians

American Academy of Pediatrics

American Medical Society for Sports Medicine

American Orthopaedic Society for Sports Medicine

American Osteopathic Academy of Sports Medicine

Preparticipation Physical Evaluation Task Force
David M. Smith, MD, FAAFP, Chair
Jeffrey R. Kovan, DO
Brent S. E. Rich, MD, ATC
Suzanne M. Tanner, MD, FAAP

Society Representatives
Stephen Hunter, MD, FACS, American Orthopaedic Society for Sports Medicine
Brent S. E. Rich, MD, ATC, American Medical Society for Sports Medicine
David M. Smith, MD, FAAFP, American Academy of Family Physicians
Suzanne M. Tanner, MD, FAAP, American Academy of Pediatrics
Leonard Wilkerson, DO, FAAFP, American Osteopathic Academy of Sports Medicine

the physician and sportsmedicine
A Division of The McGraw-Hill Companies

The Physician and Sportsmedicine
A division of the McGraw-Hill Companies
Minneapolis, New York

McGraw-Hill Healthcare
The Physician and Sportsmedicine
4530 W 77th St
Minneapolis, MN 55435
To Order: 1-800-262-4729

Project editor: Susan Hawthorne
Graphic design: Nancy Johansen-Wester
Illustration: Terry Boles, Rebekah Dodson

The Physician and Sportsmedicine

A Division of The ***McGraw-Hill*** *Companies*

Printed in the United States of America
Last digit is the print number: 9 8 7 6 5 4 3 2 1

Library of Congress Cataloging-in-Publication Data
Preparticipation physical evaluation / American Academy of Family Physicians ... [et al.] ; Preparticipation Physical Evaluation Task Force, David M. Smith, chairman ... [et al.]. — 2nd ed. p. cm. Includes bibliographical references.
ISBN 0-07-001627-5
1. Athletes—Medical examinations. I. American Academy of Family Physicians. II. Preparticipation Physical Evaluation Task Force. RC1225.P65 1996 616.07'5'088796—dc20 96-27879 CIP

PREFACE

Preparticipation Physical Evaluation, Second Edition, updates the first edition of the monograph, published in 1992. It continues to be the only publication on sports physicals endorsed by five major medical societies. We are indebted to the first edition contributing authors—John A. Lombardo, MD; James B. Robinson, MD; and David M. Smith, MD—for initiating this worthy project. In upholding their goal of making this an ongoing project with periodic updates, we are pleased to present this second edition.

Primary changes in this edition include updated clearance recommendations for various medical and musculoskeletal conditions; an expanded review of the physical examination, particularly the musculoskeletal examination; improvements to the history and physical examination forms; the addition of brief sections on alcohol and drug use, ergogenic aids, and blood-borne pathogens; recognition of the female athlete triad syndrome; and a new section discussing medicolegal considerations.

This edition of the *Preparticipation Physical Evaluation* has been reviewed more extensively than the first, and we acknowledge and greatly appreciate the excellent comments, criticisms, and suggestions of the many individuals who have reviewed specific sections or the whole document. These individuals include professional colleagues in primary care and multiple specialties, both private practitioners and academicians.

Our special thanks to society representatives Stephen Hunter, MD, and Leonard Wilkerson, DO, and to American Academy of Pediatrics Committee on Sports Medicine and Fitness members Steven J. Anderson, MD, and William L. Risser, MD, PhD, for their expertise and patience as they contributed countless hours reviewing revisions of the monograph. Their tremendous assistance and cooperation allowed timely publication of this extensive project.

And finally, we sincerely appreciate the talented editorial staff of McGraw-Hill Healthcare, and especially project editor Susan Hawthorne, for their tireless devotion in guiding this project through to completion.

David M. Smith, MD, FAAFP
Jeffrey R. Kovan, DO
Brent S. E. Rich, MD, ATC
Suzanne M. Tanner, MD, FAAP

Table *of* Contents

continued

Goals *and* Objectives

Introduction

Sports participation can enhance fitness and coordination, increase self-esteem, and provide a positive social experience for young athletes. Sometimes, though, injury or illness impedes participation. For the physician who wishes to help young athletes overcome such obstacles, or to help prevent injury or illness, the preparticipation physical evaluation (PPE) is an important tool.

This monograph guides physicians in performing the PPE for athletes of middle school, high school, or college age in either a private office setting or a station-based environment. The special concerns of athletes who have disabilities are not discussed. The monograph describes the goals of the PPE, details the history and physical examination, states clearance guidelines or refers the reader to appropriate sources, and discusses medicolegal precautions. Appropriate forms for use during the PPE are provided. It must be noted, however, that the PPE as described here has not been validated in all aspects, and, of course, new studies may call for different techniques or decisions. Examiners will therefore need to rely on their clinical judgment in PPE performance and in clearance and referral determinations.

By providing this guide, the author societies hope both to enhance the health and safety of athletes and to help make the PPE an enjoyable, informative, and useful experience for both practitioner and patient.

Goals and Objectives

The overall goal of the PPE is to help maintain the health and safety of the athlete in training and competition. Its purpose is not to exclude athletes from participation but to promote safe participation. Only 0.3% to 1.3% of athletes are denied clearance during the PPE, and only 3.2% to 13.5% require further evaluation.[1-5] If not cleared, most athletes can be redirected to another sport. The PPE is not intended to substitute for an athlete's regular health maintenance examination; however, the reality for many athletes is that the PPE will be their only health maintenance contact with a physician.

The overall goal of the PPE is achieved by adhering to its three primary objectives (table 1 and page 2).[1, 6-8] The three secondary objectives (table 1 and page 2) take advantage of the opportunity provided by physician contact with the

TABLE 1.
Objectives of the Preparticipation Physical Evaluation

Primary Objectives
Detect conditions that may predispose to injury
Detect conditions that may be life-threatening or disabling
Meet legal and insurance requirements
Secondary Objectives
Determine general health
Counsel on health-related issues
Assess fitness level for specific sports

athletes and can be fulfilled depending on available time and resources and the desires of the medical team, coaches, and athletes.

PRIMARY OBJECTIVES

(1) To detect medical or musculoskeletal conditions that may predispose an athlete to injury or illness during competition.

Such conditions include acute, recurrent, chronic, or untreated injuries or illnesses, inadequately rehabilitated injuries, and congenital or developmental problems. Early recognition of any of these minimizes time lost from play by allowing initiation of treatment. For example, an obese athlete is at an increased risk for heat illness and therefore should be advised on weight control, acclimatization, and hydration before the season starts. Similarly, an athlete with recurrent ankle sprains who has returned to sports prior to completely rehabilitating his or her ankle may require instruction or follow-up regarding appropriate rehabilitation measures.

(2) To detect potentially life-threatening or disabling medical or musculoskeletal conditions that may limit an athlete's safe participation.

Both absolute and relative contraindications are considered. For example, myocarditis is an absolute contraindication for any sport because of the risk of sudden death with exertion. Ventricular septal defect, however, is a relative contraindication because the athlete may be able to participate depending on the severity of the defect.

(3) To address legal or insurance requirements.

Each state has its own regulations concerning the medical eligibility of student-athletes. Sponsoring institutions may also have specific requirements.

SECONDARY OBJECTIVES

(1) To determine the general health of the athlete.

Although the annual PPE can be integrated into the regular examination with the athlete's personal physician, it is not meant to replace these regular examinations. However, it has been shown that for over 78% of athletes, the PPE is their only periodic health examination.[2,9] This may especially be true of athletes from low-income families who cannot afford routine medical care. Careful attention to general health maintenance, therefore, is an added benefit regardless of the setting, if time and circumstances permit.

(2) To counsel the athlete.

Depending on available time, the physician may find the opportunity during the evaluation to counsel the athlete and answer health-related questions.[6] In a busy station-based evaluation, this objective may be hard to meet, but may be attempted if this is practical or appropriate. Likewise, if the evaluation is done in the physician's office, time can be allotted if possible for this valuable service. The physician may want to explain abnormal findings more thoroughly, or discuss topics such as proper training techniques, weight control behaviors, and nutrition. Tobacco use, drinking and driving, drug use, seat belt use, prevention of sexually transmitted diseases, and birth control may also be discussed. Handouts may provide useful patient education for athletes and parents.

(3) To assess fitness level for specific sports.

Testing parameters that may affect performance or contribute to health problems or injury can be useful to athletes and coaches. The major components of fitness assessment include body composition, flexibility, strength, and endurance. Power, speed, balance, and agility also may be measured. Testing of these fitness components can establish a baseline for training and rehabilitation for the specific sport in which the athlete chooses to participate. Furthermore, the information obtained may be used as a research tool to learn more about key components of physical conditioning for specific sports.[10,11]

TIMING, SETTING, *and* STRUCTURE

QUALIFICATIONS OF THE EXAMINERS

Qualification of health care professionals to perform the PPE is based on specialty training, clinical expertise, and availability. States certify which practitioners are qualified to perform PPEs at the secondary school level; many states allow health care professionals other than physicians to perform the evaluation. At the collegiate, professional, national, and international competitive levels, the respective athletic governing bodies determine who may perform the PPE.

However, because MD/DO physicians' training allows them to deal with the broad range of problems that may be encountered during the PPE, the author societies concur that the ultimate responsibility for the PPE should ideally fall to an MD/DO physician. Physicians desiring to perform PPEs must be capable of fulfilling the goals and objectives outlined in the previous section. Primary care physicians should consult specialty physicians when a problem requires additional expertise. Conversely, if specialist physicians perform the PPE, they should consult generalists regarding issues outside their area of expertise.

Finally, under the supervision of a physician, qualified non-MD/DO health care professionals may be integrated to perform appropriate components of the evaluation (see table 2, page 6).

TIMING OF THE EVALUATION

The PPE should ideally be performed at least 6 weeks prior to preseason practice. This allows time for correction or rehabilitation of any identified problems. To avoid potential difficulties of scheduling PPEs in midsummer, evaluations may be performed at the end of the previous school year. It is the athlete's responsibility to report injuries or illnesses occurring in the interval between the PPE and the start of the season to the coach, the athletic trainer, and/or the athlete's physician.

FREQUENCY OF THE EVALUATION

Opinions vary widely as to how often the young athlete needs to be evaluated. Some advocate a PPE prior to every sport season, requiring multiple examinations per year for athletes in multiple sports.[12] In some locations, a full evaluation annually is the norm.[13] Other commentators support a complete evaluation on entering a new school level (middle school, high school, or college), followed by an interim evaluation.[14] This can be either a history and limited physical evaluation annually or an annual history reviewed by a physician and focused physical examinations only for those with abnormal findings. There is consensus that if the interim history indicates a potential problem, a physical examination and other assessment as necessary should be performed (see "Interim Evaluations" page 7).

Issues to consider in making the choice of examination frequency for a given program include (1) requirements of the school or state; (2) the degree of risk of the sport; (3) cost, especially out-of-pocket expenses for students, since these will be barriers to participation; and (4) availability of qualified personnel.

Thus, the optimal frequency of the PPE has not been established. However, the entry-level complete screening evaluation followed by a limited annual reevaluation works well in meeting the previously outlined primary objectives for the PPE.

A complete PPE should be performed annually when continuity of care is in question or there are no previous records to demonstrate prior normal examinations.

METHODS OF EVALUATION

Overview. The two most common settings for performing the PPE are in the physician's office or in a station-based screening environment.

Office-Based PPE. ***Advantages.*** Continuity of care is one of the most important advantages of having the PPE performed by the athlete's personal or primary care physician in an office setting. Any problems or abnormalities detected can be appropriately evaluated with consultations if needed, and treatment can be started.

If the physician has treated the athlete throughout his or her childhood, there is the added advantage of physician-patient familiarity. The physician will know the athlete's history and have a complete set of medical records, including family history, immunizations, and laboratory studies. This reduces the possibility that an abnormality will "fall through the cracks" and predispose an athlete to further problems. With this information, the physician is less likely to overlook something that was inadvertently or consciously omitted during completion of the preparticipation history form.

Familiarity also provides an opportunity to counsel the athlete on sensitive issues such as alcohol and drug use, birth control, and prevention of sexually transmitted diseases. Young athletes are far more willing to discuss these issues with someone they trust.

Disadvantages. First, many athletes do not have a personal or primary care physician. Some do not have access to comprehensive medical care, whereas others may consult a different specialist for every medical problem that arises.

Second, time for each examination may be limited in a busy physician's schedule. The demand for completing examinations before the season may exceed the availability of appointment times in a single physician's office.

Third, not all physicians have equal interest in or familiarity with sports and sports-related medical problems. Some physicians may not feel comfortable determining clearance for an athlete who has a particular problem or detecting conditions that may predispose the athlete to further injury or illness.

Fourth, the cost of an office visit may be prohibitively high for some athletes. Station-based examinations with physicians volunteering their time can usually be done at a lower cost.

Finally, an office-based examination may hamper communication among the physician, the coach, the athletic trainer, the athlete, and the athlete's parent(s) or guardian(s). Communication breakdowns may result in an athlete being disqualified without the coach and trainer knowing the reasons for disqualification. Conversely, the coach or trainer may be aware of an injury or condition that the athlete may not disclose for fear of being denied clearance.

Techniques. Essentially, the office-based PPE follows the same procedure as any other examination in a primary physician's office. Some of the potential disadvantages of the office-based examinations can be avoided by:

- Being knowledgeable about the demands of sports, the conditions affecting participation, and the treatments available to allow safe participation. The physician will need to include a sports-oriented history.
- Communicating with the athletic department staff and the athlete's parent(s) if

the athlete is a minor. Using standardized forms, such as the history, physical examination, and clearance forms provided on pages 47-49, may facilitate this communication.
- Considering alternative scheduling to help overcome the time limitations. For example, time may be allowed at the end of the day or after regular office hours to perform individual evaluations, or a station-type examination can be done using office personnel.

Station-Based PPE. *Advantages.* Station-based evaluations can be cost-effective and efficient. Several hundred can be performed in a few hours with the proper personnel and organization. This is especially important for athletes from low-income families and may become increasingly important in managed care environments.

Station-based evaluations can also use the skills and expertise of a variety of personnel including physicians, athletic trainers, physical therapists, exercise scientists/physiologists, dentists, and dietitians. Each has a separate station and can, under the direction of the physician in charge, perform portions of the evaluations. Nonspecialized personnel can efficiently handle routines such as sign-in, height and weight measurements, and vision checks.

Finally, station-based evaluations may encourage communication among coaches, athletes, administrators, and the medical team that cares for the athletes on a daily basis. Such communication helps foster good relationships and may improve the health care of the athletes.

Disadvantages. First, a large space and large number of participants in a station-based PPE can create a noisy and confusing environment. This may make several parts of the evaluation, especially the cardiovascular portion, difficult to perform.

Second, continuity of care may be compromised with station-based evaluations. If the evaluating physician is not the athlete's regular physician, coordinating consults and follow-up may be difficult.

Third, station-based evaluations may be limited by lack of time and privacy. Physicians may be forced to rush through the evaluation without adequate time or privacy for individual counseling.

Fourth, station-based evaluations do not always afford good communication between the evaluating physician, the athlete, and the athlete's parent(s) or guardian(s). Athletes may not understand why they were disqualified or need further evaluation, which can cause unnecessary concern for parents.

Techniques. The required elements of station-based evaluations can be accomplished in six stations (table 2). However, some physicians find it more efficient to separate the physical examination into two parts—medical and musculoskeletal—thus allowing the physicians present to concentrate on an area of expertise. The musculoskeletal screening can also be performed by other qualified medical personnel under the supervision of a physician. If sufficient numbers of physicians are present, further subdivision is also possible, typically into four stations: (1) head, eyes, ears, nose, and throat (HEENT); (2) cardiovascular/pulmonary; (3) gastrointestinal/genitourinary and dermatologic; and (4) musculoskeletal/neurologic. To help in focusing the physical examination, the completed history form should be carried by the athlete from station to station for review.

Examples of the optional stations and personnel who can manage them appear in table 2. Fitness assessments, if done, may be completed at a later time.

Several techniques can limit the potential disadvantages of station-based PPEs:
- Time limitations can be minimized by having several physicians available at once and by carefully scheduling the examinations. Using a different room for each station and maintaining an orderly flow are also helpful. Evaluations can be scheduled by time slots, and personnel can be reassigned if necessary to accommodate slower stations. This should allow enough time for thorough evaluations and help avoid a rush.
- Privacy concerns can be lessened by informing the athletes in advance of the detailed nature of the examination and requiring consistent attire for all athletes

(see page 43). If male and female athletes are present, their medical examinations should be performed in separate areas. Having a private individual counseling room for discussion of sensitive issues can maintain confidentiality and facilitate better communication with the athlete. In some settings, it is possible to provide private rooms for all examination stations.

- Familiarity and continuity of care can be enhanced in the station format by enlisting the assistance of physicians who are primary physicians for many of the students being examined.
- To facilitate follow-up, athletes who are not cleared for participation because of illness or injury should be referred to their primary physician or, if necessary, given other recommendations to assist them in clearance. Athletes from low-income families, in particular, may need help in arranging and completing follow-up evaluations. If there is a team physician, he or she should keep—and follow up on—a list of athletes who are disqualified or who require further evaluation before final clearance. One follow-up technique is to retain the clearance form until the opinion of the consulting physician is obtained.
- Communication between the evaluating physician, the team physician, the consulting physician, the coach or athletic trainer, the athlete, and the athlete's parent(s) can be enhanced by filling out the history, physical examination, and clearance forms (pages 47-49) with care. A triplicate or photocopied clearance form can allow the athlete and coach to keep copies while the physician retains the original, along with the history and physical examination forms, as an official medical record. The physician also should discuss an athlete's problem with the athlete's parent(s) or guardian(s) to ensure proper communication and alleviate any unnecessary concern if the athlete is not cleared. If the athlete is not cleared for the desired sport, the evaluating physician should counsel the athlete concerning alternate permissible activities.

TABLE 2.

Required and Optional Stations and Personnel for Station-Based Preparticipation Physical Evaluations

Required Stations	Personnel
Sign-in	Ancillary personnel (coach, nurse, community volunteer)
Height, weight	Ancillary personnel
Vital signs	Ancillary personnel
Vision	Ancillary personnel
Physical examination*	Physician*
History review, assessment and clearance	Physician
Optional Stations	**Personnel**
Nutrition	Dietitian
Dental	Dentist
Injury evaluation†	Physician
Flexibility	Athletic trainer, physical therapist
Body Composition	Athletic trainer, exercise physiologist, physical therapist
Strength	Athletic trainer, coach, exercise physiologist, physical therapist
Speed, agility, power endurance, balance	Athletic trainer, coach exercise physiologist

**The physical examination can be subdivided if more than one physician is present. See text. Qualified medical personnel may perform the musculoskeletal examination under the direction of a physician.*

†A musculoskeletal injury evaluation station may be used to provide a more complete evaluation when a musculoskeletal injury is detected during the required musculoskeletal screening examination.

INTERIM EVALUATIONS

The frequency of interim evaluations varies according to state law and other considerations (see "Frequency of the Evaluation," page 3). The purpose of the interim evaluation is to assess problems that have occurred since the athlete's full PPE. A current and complete medical history, such as that on page 47, is reviewed by a physician, who determines what parts of the physical examination should be performed. For example, an athlete who has no chronic diseases and who has had no injuries or significant illnesses during the intervening period may require only a check of blood pressure, height, and weight. An athlete who has had a lateral ankle sprain may also require examination of the ankle, including assessment of range of motion and stress testing with the anterior drawer and talar tilt tests for lateral ligament laxity. An athlete who has had an episode of dizziness or palpitations during exertion may require cardiovascular assessment.

In using the forms on pages 47-48, the athlete should complete the entire medical history form, but the evaluating physician needs only to complete the pertinent section(s) of the physical examination form.

ROUTINE SCREENING TESTS

Though issues surrounding routine laboratory screening tests are frequently discussed and oftentimes controversial, the author societies concur that routine laboratory screening tests in asymptomatic athletes should not be required for the PPE. This judgment hinges on the difference between screening and diagnostic tests. The value of a screening test or procedure depends on two variables: (1) the predictive value of the proposed screen, which is in turn affected by the prevalence of the condition in the population being screened, and (2) the ability to reduce morbidity and/or mortality by identifying the condition with the screening method. The screening test must also be acceptable in terms of cost and potential side effects. The value of a diagnostic test, on the other hand, is in its ability to pinpoint a condition for which suspicion already exists by history and/or physical examination.

When evaluating screening tests with the aforementioned criteria, studies have not supported the use of such tests as urinalysis, complete blood count, chemistry profile, lipid profile, ferritin level, or sickle cell trait in the PPE.[13,15-18] Similarly, extensive cardiopulmonary testing (eg, with electrocardiogram (ECG), echocardiogram, exercise stress testing, or spirometry) for routine screening in the PPE is not recommended.[19-25]

Authors of a recent study[26] were able to perform inexpensive echocardiograms by using donated equipment and free cardiologists' interpretations. These authors state that echocardiographic screening provides valuable information efficiently and economically. However, their low costs cannot generally be duplicated, and earlier reports have found that screening echocardiography in the PPE is not cost-effective in identifying athletes at risk for sudden death.[20-23] Furthermore, during the 2,997 examinations performed in the recent study,[26] no abnormalities were identified that precluded participation in sports.

Another area of recent research is in effective ways to screen athletes for exercise-induced asthma (EIA). With the prevalence of undiagnosed EIA in high school, collegiate, and Olympic athletes estimated at 3% to 14%,[24, 27-29] it is important to attempt to identify these athletes in the PPE. However, studies have shown that history, physical examination, and resting spirometry are not reliable in identifying athletes who have EIA.[24,25,28,30] Exercise challenge tests, which are more sensitive than history and physical examination alone, may be necessary to identify the disorder.[24,25,31] However, large, reproducible population studies with cost-benefit analysis are currently lacking. Therefore, use of routine screening exercise challenge tests as part of the PPE is not currently recommended.

Findings from the medical history or physical examination may indicate a need to arrange specific diagnostic tests. For example, a hematologic profile and ferritin level may be recommended to check for anemia or iron deficiency without anemia in an athlete who has fatigue, pallor, performance decline, heavy menstrual bleeding, low calorie intake, or avoidance of red meat in the diet. A lipid profile to test for familial hypercholesterolemia is recommended in an athlete who has a family history of premature atherosclerotic heart disease or a parent with a high cholesterol level. Urinalysis may be indicated in an athlete with dysuria, hematuria, or a family history of certain types of kidney disease. Clearance for sports participation while waiting for such tests to be performed needs individual assessment, but usually the athlete is allowed to participate in most activities.

Two specific tests—urine drug screening and human immunodeficiency virus (HIV) screening—deserve mention. Routine urine drug testing at the elite amateur and professional levels is now fairly common, whereas mandatory HIV testing is still rare, although certain boxing organizations require it.[31] Physicians performing PPEs should be aware of and carefully follow the screening test guidelines established by the athletic governing body under which the athlete competes. Physicians must also consider the medical, legal, and confidentiality issues that drug screening and HIV testing entail. Furthermore, if drug screening or HIV testing is implemented, a formal plan for secure sample collection and an institutional policy for dealing with positive tests must be established.

While mandatory testing of athletes for HIV or hepatitis is not recommended[32] voluntary testing should be encouraged for athletes with exposure to blood products, appropriate constitutional symptoms of disease, or significant risk factors detected during the PPE. Risk factors include (1) multiple sex partners, (2) sexual contact with infected individuals, (3) blood transfusions before 1985, (4) sexually transmitted diseases including hepatitis B virus, and (5) history of intravenous drug abuse or injections of ergogenic drugs, or use of such drugs by sexual partners, (6) male homosexuality, and (7) in girls, bisexual partners.[32]

The PPE Medical History

OVERVIEW

The medical history is the cornerstone of any medical evaluation. A complete history will identify approximately 75% of problems affecting athletes.[2,9] However, in one study,[9] only 39% of histories reported by athletes agreed with information given by their parent(s). In addition, illiteracy or language barriers may further diminish the yield from the medical history. To increase the information obtained, the athlete and parents should, if possible, complete the history form (page 47) together before the examination. The parents should sign the history form, and ideally the physician reviews it with the athlete before the physical examination. At times, insisting that parents sign the form may interfere with the completion of the PPE: for example, in school-based clinics or when the parents have neglected to comply.

The recommended baseline questions that follow here and on the history form emphasize the areas of greatest concern for sports participation, although several questions important to general health maintenance in the adolescent population are also included.

QUESTIONS

1. Have you had a medical illness or injury since your last checkup or sports physical?

Do you have an ongoing or chronic illness?

These questions are placed first because they help the physician by "red flagging" the most recent problems. They also help stimulate the memories of the athlete and his or her parent(s) so that a complete history can be obtained.

2. Have you ever been hospitalized overnight?

Have you ever had surgery?

These questions may reveal factors related to past or recent serious illness that could affect participation. Also, people are more likely to remember going to the hospital or having surgery than a particular diagnosis; thus, asking about these events may trigger memory of a significant problem.

The questions could also help determine whether a medical illness is under proper control. For example, an athlete who requires frequent admissions for diabetes, seizures, or exacerbations of asthma may need better medical control before competing. The surgical history is important in determining whether the athlete has had adequate time for healing and rehabilitation.

3. Are you currently taking any prescription or nonprescription (over-the-counter) medications or pills or using an inhaler?

Have you ever taken any supplements or vitamins to help you gain or lose weight or improve your performance?

Understanding the athlete's use of medication for chronic disease (insulin, anticonvulsants, cardiovascular drugs, etc) is important in assessing adequate control. A team physician can also use the information to keep the medication available for emergencies and during travel. However, it is the athlete's responsibility to keep his or her medication on hand as necessary; the examining physician should make this clear to the athlete. Also, the athletic trainer and coach can be informed of potential problems, such as hypoglycemia, and instructed on how to handle them. A history of oral contraceptive prescription is useful when evaluating menstrual irregularity, and it may open the door for discussion of sexually transmitted diseases, pregnancy, and other aspects of sexuality.

Asking specifically about nonprescription drug use is important because taking over-the-counter medications, especially nonsteroidal anti-inflammatory drugs, is common. Aspirin or other platelet-inhibiting drugs may predispose an athlete to gastritis or to increased bleeding, which could be catastrophic. Excessive intake of cold or allergy medications may predispose an athlete to heat illness or cardiac arrhythmias.

Inquiring about the use of nutritional supplements such as vitamins, minerals, amino acids, protein supplements, and other so-called ergogenic aids is important because such supplements in large doses may produce adverse effects. A pattern of taking supplements should also raise questions about use of other ergogenic aids, such as anabolic steroids.

4. Do you have any allergies (for example, to pollen, medicine, food, or stinging insects)?

Have you ever had a rash or hives develop during or after exercise?

A history of allergy to any medication (eg, penicillin, sulfa drugs, aspirin) should be obtained and noted in the record to prevent inadvertent administration of these drugs. Allergy to hymenopteran (bee, wasp, yellow jacket, fire ant) envenomation and/or a history of exercise-induced anaphylaxis or exercise-induced urticaria should be noted so that proper emergency medication (subcutaneous epinephrine) can be kept on hand. As with other medications, this is the responsibility of the athlete, but trainers or team physicians may choose to keep such medication in their kits as well. Seasonal allergies may be clues to chronic use of over-the-counter drugs. The presence of allergies may also alert the clinician to the possibility of asthma or EIA.

5. Have you ever passed out during or after exercise?

Have you ever been dizzy during or after exercise?

Have you ever had chest pain during or after exercise?

Do you get tired more quickly than your friends do during exercise?

Have you ever had racing of your heart or skipped heartbeats?

Have you had high blood pressure or high cholesterol?

Have you ever been told you have a heart murmur?

Has any family member or relative died of heart problems or a sudden death before age 50?

Have you had a severe viral infection (for example, myocarditis or mononucleosis) within the last month?[33]

Has a physician ever denied or restricted your participation in sports for any heart problems?[33]

Because over 95% of sudden deaths in athletes under age 30 are due to structural cardiac problems,[34] careful attention to the cardiovascular history is paramount. Syncope or near syncope may be a clue to underlying hypertrophic cardiomyopathy, conduction abnormalities, arrhythmias, or valve problems, such as aortic stenosis or mitral valve prolapse. Chest pain on exertion may indicate advanced atherosclerotic disease (unusual before age 30 except with abnormal lipid metabolism) or congenital abnormalities of the coronary arteries. Dyspnea on exertion may indicate structural abnormalities, valve problems, or underlying lung disease, especially exercise-induced asthma. Palpitations or skipped beats may signify arrhythmias or conduction abnormalities, such as Wolff-

Parkinson-White syndrome. Such symptoms may mandate further investigation before clearance.

A history of blood pressure elevation or heart murmur should alert the examining physician to emphasize the relevant part of the cardiovascular examination. Because several causes of sudden cardiac death may be familial (for example, hypertrophic cardiomyopathy, Marfan syndrome, and lipid abnormalities causing atherosclerotic coronary artery disease), inquiring about family cardiac history is important. Recent viral infections may lead to myocarditis, which can cause symptoms of fatigue or chest pain. Any previous disqualification from athletics because of a cardiac condition should be thoroughly investigated before a clearance decision is made.

Though athletes who abuse drugs may deny it, noting a history of anabolic steroid or cocaine use is important because these drugs have been linked to sudden cardiac death.

6. Do you have any current skin problems (for example, itching, rashes, acne, warts, fungus, or blisters)?

Review of the athlete's dermatologic history should focus primarily on infectious conditions such as herpes simplex, scabies, pubic lice, molluscum contagiosum, furunculosis, carbunculosis, and impetigo. History of any of these conditions is most important for athletes who will be involved in contact/collision sports, such as wrestling or martial arts, or in sports where spread of infection is possible through a fomite, such as a gymnastics mat, towel, or helmet. History of acne should also be included because of potential exacerbation from sweating and wearing constrictive clothing or equipment.

7. Have you ever had a head injury or concussion?

Have you ever been knocked out, become unconscious, or lost your memory?

Have you ever had a seizure?

Do you have frequent or severe headaches?

Have you ever had numbness or tingling in your arms, hands, legs, or feet?

Have you ever had a stinger, burner, or pinched nerve?

The athlete's history of any neurologic conditions or injuries, such as seizures, severe or recurrent headaches, head injuries, concussion, burners/stingers, "pinched nerves," or transient quadriplegia, deserves thorough review. It is important to note whether seizures or headaches have occurred with exercise or as a result of trauma. If the athlete has had a head injury, follow-up questions include: *Did you lose consciousness, pass out, or lose your memory? What were you told, if anything, about playing contact sports?* If the athlete has been knocked out or become unconscious, follow-up questions should be asked: *How many times? How long were you unconscious? Did you lose your memory of the event or circumstances prior to the event (retrograde amnesia)? Did you have other memory problems afterward (anterograde amnesia)? Did you have problems in the days afterward (confusion, headache, problems with schoolwork)? How long did it take you to recover? Are you still having any of these problems?* If the athlete is still having symptoms suggestive of postconcussion syndrome, consultation with a neurologist, neurosurgeon, or sports medicine physician experienced with this disorder is necessary (see page 39).

Burners/stingers and pinched nerves are traumatic injuries secondary to compression or stretching of the cervical nerve roots or brachial plexus. Signs and symptoms include unilateral numbness or tingling in an upper extremity. Transient neck pain and weakness are sometimes noted. Neurologic signs (weakness) disappear rapidly, but symptoms (paresthesias) may linger for several minutes. Rarely, however, permanent neurologic sequelae may result.[35]

Cervical spinal cord neurapraxia with transient quadriplegia is a rare entity that may result from trauma. It manifests as burning pain, numbness or tingling, and weakness or paralysis of all four extremities. Of equal concern are similar symptoms that affect bilateral upper extremities or unilateral upper and lower extremities simultaneously, as these indicate spinal cord pathology. Recovery usually is complete within 10 to 15 minutes, although some cases resolve gradually over 36 to 48 hours. Either condition may be found in individuals with cervical spine stenosis, congenital fusion, cervical instability, or intervertebral disc protrusion that decreases the anteroposterior spinal canal diameter. It is important to note that this disorder also may occur in individuals with neck trauma who do not have predisposing abnormalities.

If the athlete has had recurrent burners/stingers, transient quadriplegia, or other signs or symptoms of cervical spine pathology, the examiner should determine whether cervical spine radiographs, including flexion and extension views, or further diagnostic studies (eg, magnetic resonance imaging, myelography) have been performed and what previous recommendations have been given. Indications for further evaluation include recurrent burners/stingers, unresolved neurologic signs or symptoms, and transient quadriplegia.

Burners/stingers do not automatically preclude participation if cervical spine abnormalities (eg, cervical spine instability or degenerative changes) and evidence of permanent neurologic damage are absent. Athletes with a history of burners/stingers should be referred to coaches or athletic trainers for instruction on neck and upper extremity strengthening; proper technique, such as in tackling; and protective measures such as wearing properly fitted shoulder pads or a neck roll.

8. Have you ever become ill from exercising in the heat?

Because heat disorders are often recurrent, review and documentation of an athlete's history of heat-related disorders is extremely important, especially if he or she is training or competing in a hot and/or humid environment. Problems such as frequent heat-associated muscle cramps, heat exhaustion, and difficulty acclimatizing to heat should be reviewed. If the athlete is taking medications or supplements that may increase the risk of heat-related disorders (eg, antihistamines, caffeine, or psychomotor stimulants, such as methylphenidate or methamphetamines), the examiner should check whether these could be eliminated during hot and humid months. Appropriate monitoring of pre- and post-exercise weight may demonstrate a need for rehydration before the next exercise session. Also, counseling regarding frequent fluid replacement is suggested.

9. Do you cough, wheeze, or have trouble breathing during or after activity?
Do you have asthma?
Do you have seasonal allergies that require medical treatment?

An attempt to identify athletes who have asthma or EIA should be made during the PPE. They may need additional medical treatment in certain situations, such as in cold weather or during allergy seasons. Identification and treatment can allow individuals with EIA to train and compete effectively and avoid being labeled as "out of shape" or "loafers."

10. Do you use any special protective or corrective equipment or devices that aren't usually used for your sport or position (for example, knee brace, special neck roll, foot orthotics, retainer on your teeth, hearing aid)?

Because athletes and their parents may forget about a particular problem, it is helpful to inquire about the use of special equipment. Often a special pad or brace will alert the physician to a problem. Examples include an athlete who uses a knee brace to "protect" a previously injured knee, and a football player who uses a special neck roll for recurrent brachial plexus injury. The physician may choose to evaluate the status of the equipment and, if necessary, suggest replacement, discontinuance, or alternatives. If the equipment has been ordered by another physician, it is generally best to discuss it with that physician before suggesting a change. Asking about mouth guards may be unnecessary as they are now required in most collision sports. However, mouth guards are recommended for all athletes who have braces on their teeth.

11. Have you had any problems with your eyes or vision?
Do you wear glasses, contacts, or protective eyewear?

With this question, the examiner is specifically looking for athletes who are "functionally one eyed" (a term developed by the American Academy of Ophthalmology) because their best corrected vision is poorer than 20/40 in one eye. It is also important to obtain a history of eye injury or surgery. If the athlete wears glasses or eye guards, it is important to ensure that the lenses and frames are safe for the sport in which they are used.[36]

12. Have you ever had a sprain, strain, or swelling after injury?
Have you broken or fractured any bones or dislocated any joints?
Have you had any other problems with pain or swelling in muscles, tendons, bones, or joints?

In reviewing the history of the musculoskeletal system, the examining physician should focus on any history of injury to bones, such as acute fracture or stress fracture; to joints or ligaments, such as dislocation, subluxation, instability, or sprain; and to muscles or tendons, such as contusion, hematoma, strain, or tendinitis.

The treatment the athlete received for each injury should be reviewed, including both conservative and operative treatment. In addition, the physician should note any specific rehabilitation program provided, including type and duration of exercise therapy and physical modalities. Finally, the examiner should determine whether the athlete was declared fully rehabilitated by the treating physician or therapist and what recommendations were given to maintain strength and flexibility. Updated records from referring physicians, therapists, or other medical personnel may benefit the physician in making clearance decisions at a later time.

In athletes with unresolved musculoskeletal pain and swelling after an injury, diagnostic radiography may be warranted to exclude occult fracture, growth plate abnormalities, or osteochondritis dissecans. In the absence of trauma, recurrent joint swelling and pain may require further diagnostic work-up with attention to rheumatologic disorders.

13. Do you want to weigh more or less than you do?
Do you lose weight regularly to meet weight requirements for your sport?

Because of the ever-growing concern about the prevalence of disordered eating in the adolescent and athletic population, attention to athletes' perceptions of their weight and their weight-control behaviors is imperative. The term *disordered eating* includes a range of unhealthy nutritional behaviors including inadvertent calorie deprivation (ie, poor nutritional habits), self-induced vomiting, laxative use, diuretic use, anorexia nervosa, and bulimia nervosa. Disordered eating may be most prevalent in athletes participating in sports with weight classes (eg, wrestling, rowing, judo), sports in which judging may be influenced by appearance (eg, gymnastics, figure skating, diving), and sports emphasizing leanness for optimal performance (eg, track and field, distance running).[37] The disorders are most common in female athletes (10:1).[38]

If a nonobese athlete reports a desired weight that is much lower than his or her actual weight, further questions should be pursued, such as: *How much would you like to weigh? In the last year what was your highest weight? Lowest weight? Have you ever tried diet pills, sitting in a sauna, diuretics, laxatives, vomiting, or similar techniques to lose weight?* Analysis of dietary habits and food preferences may require referral to a dietitian or nutritionist. Abnormalities detected during the physical examination may occasionally include the stigmata of anorexia nervosa or bulimia nervosa; namely, oral ulcerations, decreased tooth enamel, bradycardia, skin changes (eg, hirsutism, dry and coarse texture), hypothermia, hypotension, and edema.

An athlete who has an eating disorder, however, may falsely deny using pathologic weight-control methods. Fears of restricted athletic participation, loss of self-control, and uncovering of underlying personal stressors may make athletes leery of providing accurate information. It is essential that the examiner be direct yet supportive in questioning the athlete. Confidentiality is required.

Historical data regarding menstrual history, stress fracture, dietary habits, medication abuses, and excessive exercise may alert the examiner to the recently recognized female athlete triad (interrelated disordered eating, amenorrhea, and osteopenia). To uncover excessive exercise the follow-up question *What exercise do you do in addition to training for your sport?* can be used.

Treatment of eating disorders or the female athlete triad requires a team of professionals, including a dietitian, psychotherapist, and physician familiar with the management of this difficult entity. Therefore, referral of the athlete to his or her primary care provider for planning of such care may be indicated.

An athlete who reports a sudden weight increase, or who indicates a desired weight that greatly exceeds his or her actual weight, may be using or at risk for using anabolic steroids.

It may be appropriate to provide an estimated realistic ideal weight range and proper nutrition guidance at a follow-up appointment.

14. Do you feel stressed out?

An affirmative response about stress is a good general indicator of existing or potential psychosocial problems. Many teens engage in health-threatening behaviors, such as use of tobacco, alcohol, performance-enhancing agents, and "recreational" drugs, or having unprotected sex. Others have significant family or school problems. Although only some of these behaviors, such as cocaine use, are directly relevant to safe sports participation, the examiner may take advantage of the contact offered by the PPE to discuss these important concerns if time or circumstances permit.

Most young athletes will hesitate to respond in writing to detailed questions about drug use, weight or eating problems, sexuality, or their home or school situation, especially if their parents review and sign the form. However, they may be willing to discuss these issues with the examining physician during the PPE. Therefore, it is recommended that questions about these issues be asked verbally as follow-ups to the general question about stress. Another approach is to ask a more general follow-up question such as *Do you feel you get the support you need to deal with this stress?* This may allow an evaluation of the home situation and the family support system. Alternatively, a question such as *Do you have any other concerns you would like to discuss?* may provide an opening for a discussion of sensitive issues.

Health-threatening behaviors of particular concern—which team physicians can watch for and educate their patient-athletes about—are alcohol or drug abuse and activities that can spread blood-borne pathogens.

Alcohol and drug abuse. The use of illicit drugs and alcohol is prevalent in American society. Athletes are at risk, just as nonathletes are.

Alcohol. Alcohol has significant effects on the neurologic, endocrine, and hematopoietic systems, as well as on the liver, where it is primarily metabolized. Adverse performance effects include impairment in aerobic metabolism and decreases in balance, fine motor coordination, hand-eye coordination, visual tracking, and reaction time. Also, the risk of motor vehicle accidents increases with alcohol consumption. Finally, this drug is addictive, leading to chronic dependence.

Illicit drug use. "Street" or "pleasure" drugs, including but not limited to marijuana, cocaine/crack, heroin, amphetamines, barbiturates, LSD, and PCP, are illegal and their use does not accord with the ethical principles of athletic competition; nor do such drugs aid performance.

Tobacco products. Cigarette smoking is a significant cause of lung cancer, chronic bronchitis, emphysema, cataracts, and other diseases. Smokeless tobacco causes oral cancer and other mouth disorders. Chronic use of either form of tobacco results in nicotine addiction.

The National Collegiate Athletic Associationd (NCAA) bans the use of tobacco products by student-athletes and game personnel during practice and competition because of their harmful health effects, but the United States Olympic Committee (USOC) does not ban tobacco, since it does not enhance performance. Because smoking negatively affects oxygen utilization and heart rate and delays healing of fractures, performance may also be diminished. Nicotine ingested from smokeless tobacco does not improve response time.[39,40]

Ergogenic aids. Ergogenic aids are drugs, techniques, substances, or devices used to enhance performance. They range from hazardous substances, such as anabolic steroids and recombinant erythropoietin, to benign forms of dietary manipulation. The objective in using them is to gain a competitive advantage. The PPE may provide, time permitting, an avenue for giving sound advice about proper training and nutrition and educating athletes about the side effects of ergogenic aid use.

Anabolic steroids include testosterone and its synthetic derivatives. They promote anabolic (protein building) and androgenic (masculinizing) activity. They may be taken orally or be injected. Side effects linked to anabolic steroid use include liver damage, testicular atrophy, gynecomastia, menstrual cycle irregularities, hirsutism, changes in libido, acne, increases in LDL cholesterol, and premature closure of the growth plates in long bones; additionally, anabolic steroid use has been associated with sudden cardiac death.[41] Of note, anabolic steroid use is banned by the NCAA, USOC, and many other sports organizations.

The goals of ingesting nutritional supplements and manipulating diet are to prevent fatigue, increase energy stores, establish competitive body weight, and facilitate the body's biochemical reactions. Carbohydrate loading and ingestion of vitamins, minerals, amino acids, or electrolyte solutions are examples of these techniques.[32]

Blood-borne illness. If time permits, the PPE may be effectively used to educate athletes about blood-borne pathogens, particularly HIV and hepatitis B virus (HBV), in an age-appropriate manner. Such efforts can also be continued by appropriately trained school personnel. Suggested teaching points include (1) sexual transmission of these diseases will be prevented by abstinence and reduced by limiting the number of sexual partners and by condom use; (2) needles (sometimes used to inject illicit drugs or ergogenic agents, such as anabolic steroids) should never be shared; (3) athletes should not share such personal items as water bottles, toothbrushes, razors, and nail clippers.

Mandatory testing for blood-borne pathogens is not recommended,[32] but voluntary testing should be encouraged for those at high risk for infection (see "Routine Screening Tests" on page 7).

15. Record the dates of your most recent immunizations (shots) for tetanus _________, measles ________, hepatitis B _________, and chickenpox _________.

Although delinquent immunizations do not disqualify an athlete from sports, immunization status is an important health maintenance concern that can be quickly assessed during the PPE. If an athlete is not up-to-date on immunizations, the physician can help plan an appointment and follow up as appropriate.

The booster dose of tetanus and diphtheria toxoid adsorbed for adult use (Td), previously recommended between ages 14 and 16 years, may now be given between ages 11 and 12 years with the second dose of the measles-mumps-rubella (MMR) vaccine.[42] The Centers for Disease Control and Prevention (CDC)[42] recommends that Td toxoid then be given every 10 years unless there is an earlier need for wound management.[43]

The CDC recommends that children receive their first dose of the MMR vaccine at age 12 to 15 months, followed by a second dose between ages 4 and 6 years or between ages 11 and 12 years.[42] Repeat vaccination may be considered when an individual enters college if a recent measles outbreak has occurred or if the college requires a preentrance immunization.

One dose of varicella vaccine is recommended between ages 11 and 12 years if the vaccine has not been received previously and if there is no documented previous infection with varicella.[43] After age 12, a second dose of varicella vaccine is administered 4 to 8 weeks after the initial dose.

Implementation of HBV immunization for infants began in 1991, so most adolescents are not yet immunized. The CDC[44] recommends that infants 18 months or younger and all adolescents should routinely receive the three-dose series. Children between 19 months and adolescence may also be immunized, but this does not need to be done routinely. The pediatric dose of the vaccine can be used with the same effectiveness up to age 19 at a substantial savings over use of the adult dose. Special efforts should be made to vaccinate high-risk patients.

16. (Females only)
When was your first menstrual period?
When was your most recent menstrual period?
How much time do you usually have from the start of one period to the start of another?
How many periods have you had in the last year?
What was the longest time between periods in the last year?

A detailed menstrual history is important. Amenorrhea, both primary and secondary, should be detected by history. Primary amenorrhea is defined as the absence of menarche at age 16. Secondary amenorrhea refers to missing at least three consecutive menstrual periods in a previously menstruating female; the most common cause is pregnancy. Athletes with amenorrhea or oligomenorrhea (ie, periods that occur at intervals greater than every 35 days) should be referred to their primary care physician or to a gynecologist for further evaluation. A search for other causes of menstrual disturbance, such as pregnancy, should be undertaken before attributing amenorrhea to the female athlete triad (see pages 13 and 37) or to excessive exercise. Problems that may accompany exercise-associated amenorrhea include poor nutrition, inadequate bone mineralization, and stress fractures.

The physician may also inquire about recent Pap tests in women who are over age 18 or who are sexually active, and advise the athlete to see her personal physician for health maintenance, Pap testing, and instruction in breast self-examination.

THE PPE *Physical* EXAMINATION

OVERVIEW

The PPE physical examination is a screening tool emphasizing the areas of greatest concern in sports participation and areas identified as problems in the history. Males should be dressed in shorts and females in shorts and tank tops to facilitate an adequate examination. Table 3 lists the components of the physical examination. The form on page 48 can be used for the complete or interim (page 7) preparticipation physical examinations.

HEIGHT AND WEIGHT

Height and weight are measured and recorded. Extremely thin individuals may warrant questioning about recent weight loss, eating habits, or body image. Referral for further evaluation is indicated if an eating disorder or growth disturbance is suspected. Obese athletes can be referred for counseling on diet, exercise, and behavior modification for weight control.

Determination of body composition with skinfold calipers or other devices is an optional component of the PPE. It may allow estimation of ideal weight range in sports requiring weight control, such as wrestling, or in obese or thin athletes. It is difficult, however, to predict the exact ideal percentage of body fat for a participant in a given sport.

TABLE 3.
Standard Components of the Preparticipation Physical Examination

Height

Weight

Eyes
- Visual acuity (Snellen chart)
- Differences in pupil size

Oral Cavity

Ears

Nose

Lungs

Cardiovascular System
- Blood pressure
- Pulses (radial, femoral)
- Heart (rate, rhythm, murmurs)

Abdomen
- Masses
- Tenderness
- Organomegaly

Genitalia (males only)
- Single or undescended testicle
- Testicular mass
- Hernia

Skin
- Rashes
- Lesions

Musculoskeletal System
- Contour, range of motion, stability, and symmetry of neck, back, shoulder/arm, elbow/forearm, wrist/hand, hip/thigh, knee, leg/ankle, foot

HEAD, EYES, EARS, NOSE AND THROAT

Visual acuity, measured with a standard Snellen eye chart, should be 20/40 or better in each eye, with or without corrective lenses. Athletes who have absence of one eye, best corrected vision poorer than 20/40 in either eye, or a history of significant eye injury or surgery will need appropriate eye protection if they wish to participate in sports that have a high risk of eye injury (see page 35). If the athlete already has protective eyewear, this should be checked to ensure that it is in good condition and is of the appropriate type (see page 36).

The pupils should be examined for anisocoria (unequal size). Although many normal people have a slight difference in pupil size (physiologic anisocoria), a marked difference in pupil size occasionally may be noted in otherwise normal eyes. Awareness of this baseline anisocoria is important in the event of a head injury, when comparison with the athlete's usual pupil size is imperative. Communicating this information to the athlete's trainer and/or coach is important since the examining physician or examination record may not be present at all practices and games.

The remainder of the HEENT examination assesses general well-being of these areas. The clinician should be alert to oral ulcers, gingival atrophy, and decreased enamel seen with disordered eating behaviors, especially bulimia; leukoplakia seen with smokeless tobacco use; a high-arched palate in athletes with other characteristics of Marfan syndrome; corrective braces on the teeth that may require use of a mouth guard to prevent laceration in the event of oral trauma; scarring of the tympanic membrane or auditory canals related to prior tympanostomy tube or prior infection (if indicated, a hearing screen should be performed); perforated tympanic membranes in athletes competing in water sports who would need protective earplugs; and adenopathy that may suggest malignancy or infection. Nasal polyps or a deviated septum do not affect clearance but can be identified and referred for correction.

CARDIOVASCULAR SYSTEM

Evaluation of blood pressure, using an appropriately sized cuff (large athletes may require a thigh cuff for the arm), should be completed and the measurement recorded. If blood pressure is elevated initially, repeat measurements should be taken in a few minutes and again, if necessary, after the athlete lies down and rests for 10 to 15 minutes. If the athlete's blood pressure is still elevated according to the criteria in table 4, he or she should be questioned about the use of stimulants (caffeine, nicotine, ephedrine). The condition should then be further evaluated by the athlete's primary care physician.

Palpation of the radial and femoral pulses and auscultation of the heart constitute the remainder of the cardiovascular examination. Palpation of the radial pulse is usually adequate to determine whether heart rate and rhythm are regular. Nonpalpable femoral artery pulses suggest coarctation of the aorta.

Auscultation of the heart should be performed with the athlete in the supine and standing positions.[45] Standing is preferred to sitting because the murmur of hypertrophic cardiomyopathy tends to be louder when the patient is standing. Particular attention should be paid to the presence and character of any murmurs, the timing of murmurs in relation to S1 and S2, extra heart sounds (S3, S4), and clicks. Auscultatory effects of mitral valve prolapse include a midsystolic click and sometimes a late-systolic murmur.

Various maneuvers, such as squat-to-stand, deep inspiration, or Valsalva's maneuver, can help clarify murmur type. Squatting increases venous return to the heart, which in turn increases left ventricular blood volume, stroke volume, and systemic vascular resistance. Returning to a standing position reverses these changes. Valsalva's maneuver has the opposite effects by decreasing venous return to the heart. With hypertrophic cardiomyopathy (HCM), therefore, squatting decreases the outflow obstruction and decreases the intensity of the murmur, while Valsalva increases the obstruction and increases the murmur. The harsh, systolic murmur of aortic stenosis, on the other hand, increases with squatting and decreases with Valsalva. The intensity of innocent murmurs also increases with squatting and decreases with Valsalva, but an innocent murmur can be distinguished from an aortic stenosis murmur by volume, location, duration, quality, and radiation.

In short, murmurs in adolescents are common, but any systolic murmur grade 3/6 in severity or more, any diastolic murmur, and any murmur that gets louder with Valsalva should be further evaluated before an athlete is cleared to play. If there is any uncertainty about the nature of the murmur or there are any cardiac symptoms noted in the history, referral to a cardiologist for appropriate evaluation is recommended. Also, it must be remembered that the physical examination and auscultation alone cannot detect all cases and/or types of heart disease.

Arrhythmias found on examination may require electrocardiographic evaluation to determine their specific nature. The disappearance of irregular beats with exercise usually indicates a benign condition in a structurally normal heart. If there are multifocal premature ventricular contractions, doublets, or triplets, the athlete should be examined by a cardiologist.

TABLE 4.

Classification of Hypertension by Age-Group

Age-Group (yrs)	Significant Hypertension (mm Hg)	Severe Hypertension (mm Hg)
Children (6-9)	Systolic BP ≥122 Diastolic BP ≥78	Systolic BP ≥130 Diastolic BP ≥ 86
Children (10-12)	Systolic BP ≥126 Diastolic BP ≥82	Systolic BP ≥134 Diastolic BP ≥ 90
Adolescents (13-15)	Systolic BP ≥136 Diastolic BP ≥86	Systolic BP ≥144 Diastolic BP ≥ 92
Adolescents (16-18)	Systolic BP ≥142 Diastolic BP ≥92	Systolic BP ≥150 Diastolic BP ≥ 98

Reprinted with permission from Report of the Second Task Force on Blood Pressure Control in Children—1987. Task Force on Blood Pressure Control in Children. National Heart, Lung, and Blood Institute, Bethesda, Maryland. Pediatrics 1987;79(1):1-25

In athletes who may have structural heart disease, the standard evaluation generally includes a history and physical, 12-lead ECG, echocardiogram, and exercise treadmill test. Evaluation beyond these tests usually requires the expertise of an experienced cardiologist. The 26th Bethesda Conference guidelines[46] are an excellent resource for the primary care physician concerning the cardiovascular work-up and clearance for play.

LUNGS

Pulmonary examination should reveal clear breath sounds. Pathologic findings such as wheezes or rubs may be further evaluated at a later time. If the athlete smells of tobacco, a discussion regarding tobacco use may be in order. A normal examination does not exclude EIA.

ABDOMEN

The abdomen examination should be performed with the athlete supine. The anterior superior iliac spines should be exposed to ensure adequate inspection and palpation of all four quadrants. Abdominal masses, tenderness, rigidity, or enlargement of the liver or spleen requires further evaluation prior to clearance. Occasionally, an abnormal kidney may be identified by abdomen examination, again requiring further evaluation. Female athletes should be evaluated for pregnancy by palpation for a gravid uterus in the midline from the xyphoid process to the symphysis pubis.

GENITALIA

The male genitourinary examination should focus on testicular presence or absence, undescended testicles, testicular irregularities or masses, and inguinal herniation. Counseling concerning participation in contact/collision sports is required for athletes with unpaired or undescended testicles, as discussed on page 41. Inguinal hernias should be evaluated on an individual basis.

Testicular cancer is the leading cause of cancer deaths in men 18 to 35 years of age. The PPE provides an opportunity, time permitting, to introduce the important health maintenance practice of testicular self-examination. The examining physician can advise the athlete to see his physician for instructions. For athletes who do not have a personal physician, verbal instructions or a patient handout on testicular self-examination may be provided at the time of the physical examination.

The genitourinary examination in female athletes is not part of the PPE. If warranted on the basis of the athlete's medical history, it should be deferred to a separate time and place.

The usefulness of physical maturity assessment by Tanner staging during the PPE is controversial. Proponents of Tanner staging believe that separating athletes according to stage of development may reduce injury rates in contact/collision sports, and suggest that athletes of lower Tanner stage can compete more often if separated, thus deriving psychological benefits.[47] However, others have noted that injury rates are greater in athletes of higher Tanner stage,[48] and that there is no definitive data supporting either the injury-reduction or psychological claims. Currently, Tanner staging is not used to make a decision about an athlete's participation. Therefore, the author societies no longer recommend Tanner staging as a routine part of the PPE.

SKIN

Whether in an office-based or station-based examination setting, the skin should be inspected at a consistent point in the physical examination. Attention should be given to rashes, infections, and infestations. These include eczema, impetigo, furuncles/carbuncles, herpes simplex lesions, molluscum contagiosum, fungal infections, scabies, and louse infestations. A thorough search for abnormal nevi is not possible within the limits of the PPE; however, suspicious nevi noted during the examination should be further evaluated. These should not preclude clearance for participation.

MUSCULOSKELETAL SYSTEM

The type and extent of the musculoskeletal examination appropriate for the PPE is a much-debated topic, and few data are available to guide the clinician. Examiners need to determine which method best suits a given situation, depending on history of injury, musculoskeletal signs or symptoms, resources and time available, type of sport or activity in which the athlete will participate, and the level of expertise of the examiner.

The yield of any type of musculoskeletal examination is low in asymptomatic athletes who have no history of injury. In addition, history alone has been shown to be 92% sensitive in detecting significant musculoskeletal injuries.[49] Therefore, a reasonable approach is to use a general screening examination (at right) for asymptomatic athletes who have no previous injury. If the athlete has (1) a previous injury or (2) pain, joint instability, locking, weakness, atrophy, or other signs or symptoms detected by the general screening examination or the history, the general screen should be supplemented with relevant elements of the joint-specific examination (see page 21), or the athlete should be referred to a specialist for evaluation. Alternatively, when time and resources permit, it is also reasonable to perform the entire joint-specific examination instead of a general screening examination, or to perform a sport-specific examination (see page 25).

General screening examination. General screens may be used to quickly assess joint range of motion, gross muscle strength, and muscle asymmetry, and to identify significant injuries.[49] The general screening examination described here (figure 1[13, 50]) is an adaptation of the 13-point musculoskeletal screening examination discussed in the first edition of this monograph.[13] The author societies now recommend that assessment of back extension be included in the screening examination because it may help identify spondylolysis or spondylolisthesis.

In using the general screen, however, clinicians must be aware that it does not allow determination of a specific diagnosis or severity of musculoskeletal injury. For example, it does not assess the degree of instability of a shoulder with glenohumeral joint laxity, and may not allow detection of rotator cuff injuries. Examiners must therefore supplement the general screening examination with relevant elements of the joint-specific examination when indicated by findings in the history or general screen, or they must refer the athlete to a specialist for evaluation. For example, if the history indicates past or current ankle injury or pain, or the patient is unable to perform the "duck walk" or toe raise, instability of the lateral ankle should be evaluated by anterior drawer and talar tilt testing.

Joint-specific testing. Assessing individual joints by inspection, palpation, and maneuvers well established in the literature is more definitive than the general screening examination. It may also be better suited than the sport-specific examination (see page 25) to multisport athletes. However, joint-specific examinations are more time-consuming than the general screen, may exceed the expertise of the examiner, and have a low yield in an asymptomatic athlete without a previous injury. The author societies therefore do not consider it necessary to perform the entire joint-specific examination for every athlete. Instead, portions of the examination are used as indicated by the history and findings on the general screen. However, because of its accuracy, some sports medicine practitioners prefer to use the entire joint-specific examination as their primary evaluation tool during the musculoskeletal portion of the PPE.

The complete joint-specific screening examination includes inspection and range-of-motion testing of the neck, spine, shoulders, elbows, wrists, fingers, hips, knees, ankles, and feet. Stability of the shoulders, elbows, knees, and ankles is also assessed. Symmetry of joint appearance and motion should be noted.

If the joint-specific screening examination confirms a problem, a more thorough and focused examination with relevant diagnostic testing may be indicated prior to sports clearance. If the setting and examiner expertise allow, this may be done at the time of screening.

Spine. The cervical spine should be inspected for posture and alignment. Forward flexion of the neck should allow the chin to touch the manubrium, extension should allow skyward gaze, rotation should let the chin almost touch the clavicle in either direction, and the ears should approach the shoulders on lateral flexion. Any asymmetries or deficiencies should be noted.

Examination of the thoracolumbar spine focuses on appreciating deformities. The scapulae should be level, symmetric, and flat against the chest wall. Presence or absence of scoliosis should be observed, as well as the degree of kyphosis at the thoracic level and lordosis at the lumbar level. Presence of rotatory deformities should be noted as the athlete bends forward at the waist (figure 2); pain or restriction of motion on forward flexion may indicate lumbar disc disease. Back extension should also be assessed; pain may increase in the presence of spondylolysis, spondylolisthesis, or a strain.

Upper extremity. The shoulder examination begins with inspection for symmetry with the athlete in the standing position. Range of motion in abduction (figure 3a), flexion (figure 3b), and internal and external rotation (figures 3c-d) are then assessed. The condition of the rotator cuff is tested with the "empty can test" (figure 4a), by manual resistance to internal and external rotation (figure 4b), and by eliciting any impingement sign (figure 4c). Deltoid strength is assessed by manual resistance to straight abduction (figure 5). A screen for multidirectional instability includes subluxation tests in the anterior and posterior planes in the supine athlete (figures 6a-b),

Figure 1.
The general musculoskeletal screening examination consists of the following: (1) Inspection, athlete standing, facing toward examiner (symmetry of trunk, upper extremities); (2) Forward flexion, extension, rotation, lateral flexion of neck (range of motion, cervical spine); (3) Resisted shoulder shrug (strength, trapezius); (4) Resisted shoulder abduction (strength, deltoid); (5) Internal and external rotation of shoulder (range of motion, glenohumeral joint); (6) Extension and flexion of elbow (range of motion, elbow); (7) Pronation and supination of elbow (range of motion, elbow and wrist); (8) Clench fist, then spread fingers (range of motion, hand and fingers); (9) Inspection, athlete facing away from examiner (symmetry of trunk, upper extremities); (10) Back extension, knees straight (spondylolysis/ spondylolisthesis); (11) Back flexion with knees straight, facing toward and away from examiner (range of motion, thoracic and lumbosacral spine; spine curvature; hamstring flexibility); (12) Inspection of lower extremities, contraction of quadriceps muscles (alignment, symmetry); (13) "Duck walk" four steps (motion of hip, knee, and ankle; strength; balance); (14) Standing on toes, then on heels (symmetry, calf; strength; balance).

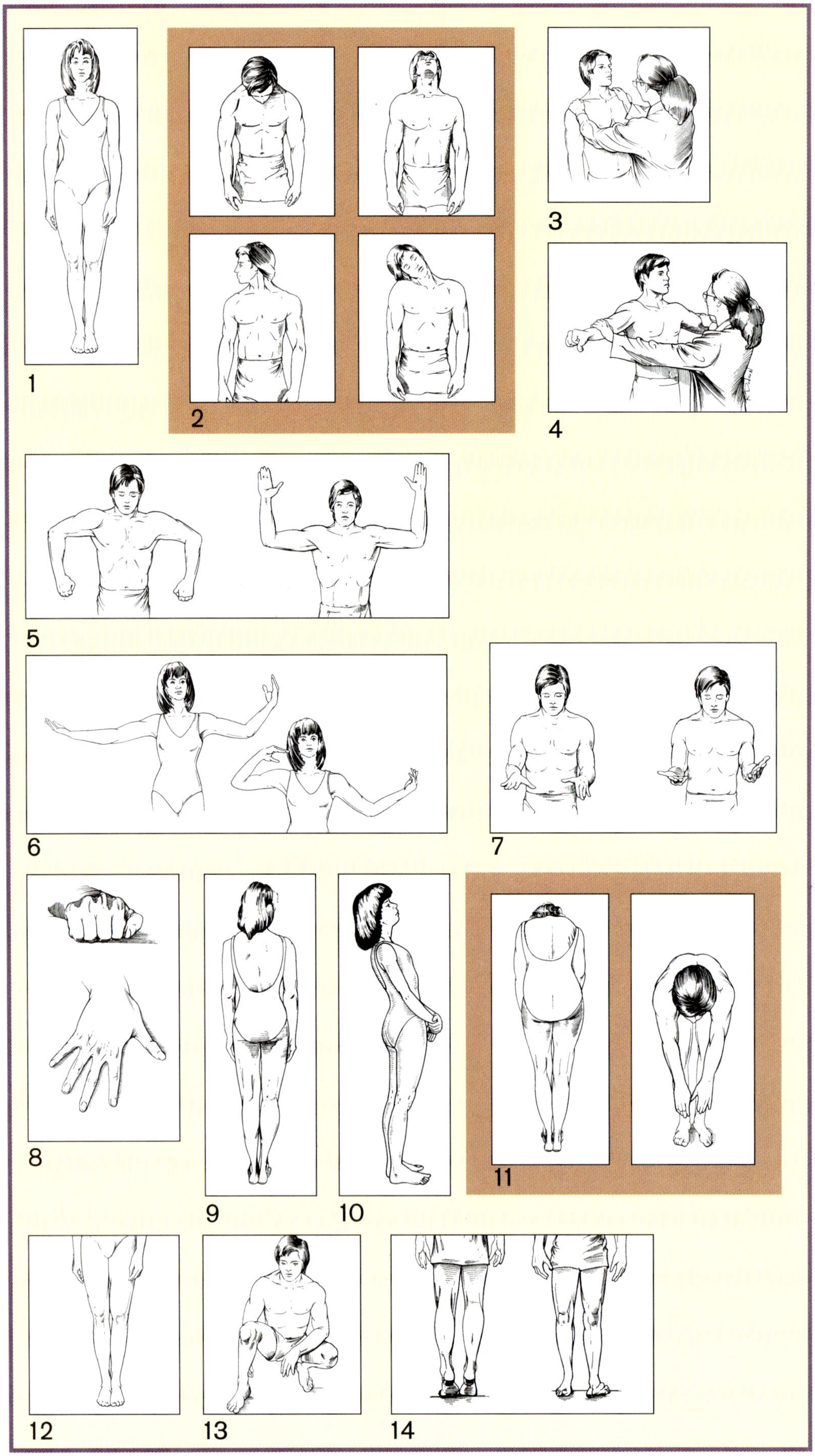

and in the inferior plane in the seated athlete (figure 6c).

The elbow is observed for swelling, discoloration, and cubital angle (figure 7). The elbow should extend fully and then flex to allow the athlete to touch the ipsilateral shoulder with the hand. Forearm motion is assessed by having the athlete pronate and supinate the forearms with the elbows bent 90° at his or her sides. The athlete should be able to turn the hand completely palm up and completely palm down.

The hand and wrist are evaluated for symmetry. Wrists should palmar flex equally to about 80° and dorsiflex to 70° or more. There should be more ulnar deviation than radial deviation. The fingers should be able to close into a full fist, and each fingernail should point at the scaphoid bone with the fingers flexed across the palm. Intrinsic muscle function can be checked by having the athlete touch each fingertip with the thumb and spread and close the extended fingers.

Lower extremity. The hip examination begins with observation of the standing posture. Iliac crest height should be level and the athlete should be able to stand on each foot without any tilting of the pelvis. Hip range of motion can be assessed with the athlete lying supine. With the hip in neutral and the knee extended, the hip joint is rotated internally and externally (a "log roll" movement), and any asymmetry is noted. Symmetry of abduction and adduction should also observed. Hip flexion should be beyond 90°, and the knees should come straight toward the chest; any external rotation indicates an intrinsic hip deformity. With the hip and knee flexed to 90°, the hip joint is rotated again (figure 8). Keeping the athlete's hip flexed 90° and extending the knee checks hamstring flexibility. The popliteal angle should be 0° to 10°.

With the athlete standing, inspection should reveal a normal leg-thigh valgus angulation of 12° or less in males and 18° or less in females. The patella should be observed for an abnormal lateral or alta position with the athlete seated. The remainder of the knee examination should be performed on both knees with the athlete supine. Each patella should be evaluated for hypermobility by translating the patella medially and laterally with the knee in 30° of flexion; comparison with the opposite side should be made. Joint line tenderness may indicate a meniscal tear. Any amount of knee effusion should be noted. Knee range of motion should be from full extension to approximately 140° of flexion. Knee ligament stability tests include the Lachman test for anterior cruciate ligament deficiency (figure 9a); anterior and posterior drawer tests (figures 9b-c) for anterior and posterior cruciate ligament insufficiencies, respectively; and varus and valgus stress tests for collateral ligament laxities (figure 9d-e).

The ankles are evaluated for normal appearance with the athlete first standing, then sitting. In the seated position, active dorsiflexion to 20° and plantar flexion to 40° should be present. With the knee extended, tightness in the Achilles tendon can be assessed by passively dorsiflexing the seated athlete's ankle while observing the lateral aspect of the leg and ankle. The ankle should dorsiflex 15° to 20° past neutral. Stress testing for lateral ligament laxity includes the anterior drawer test for anterior subluxation (figure 10a) and the talar tilt test for lateral ligament stability (figure 10b).

On inspection of the foot, cavus or rigid

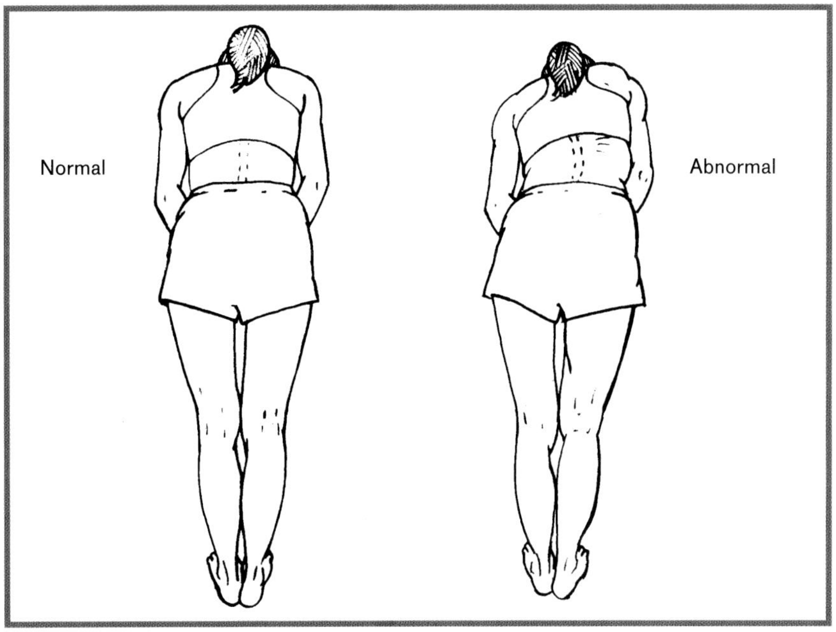

Figures 2-10: Terry Boles

Figure 2.
As part of the thoracolumbar spine examination, the athlete bends forward at the waist. The rotatory deformities of scoliosis, such as asymmetrical, prominent ribs, curvature of the spine, and/or an asymmetrical waist, are accentuated in this position.

Figure 3.
Shoulder range of motion is evaluated in four directions. In abduction (a) and forward flexion (b), the athlete should be able to reach completely overhead without excessive or asymmetrical motion of the scapula; in internal rotation (c), the fingertips should reach approximately to the bottom of the opposite scapula; and in external rotation (d), the fingertips should approach the top of the opposite scapula.

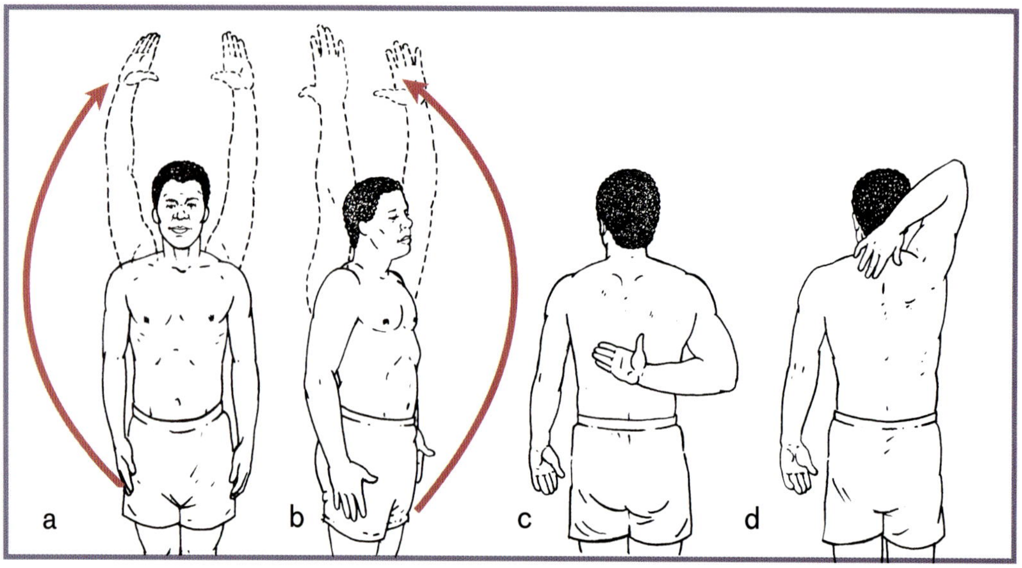

Figure 4.
Rotator cuff function can be evaluated with several tests. The "empty can test" (a) isolates the supraspinatus muscle: The patient places both shoulders in 60° to 90° abduction and 30° forward flexion with thumbs down, and the examiner resists further abduction. At 90° abduction, manual resistance to internal and then external rotation (b) may reveal weakness or pain in the presence of rotator cuff dysfunction. To detect impingement, the physician fully abducts and internally rotates the athlete's shoulder (c) and notes exacerbation of shoulder pain.

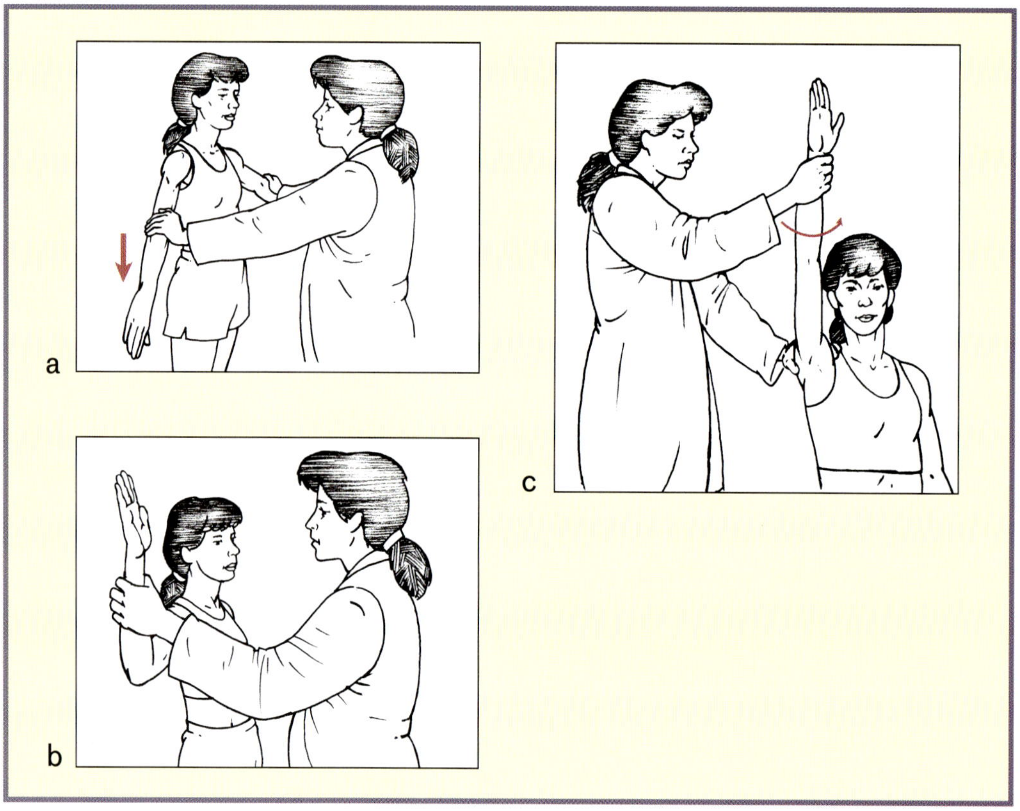

Figure 5.
Deltoid strength can be assessed by manually resisting straight abduction of the arm. Comparison for symmetry is important.

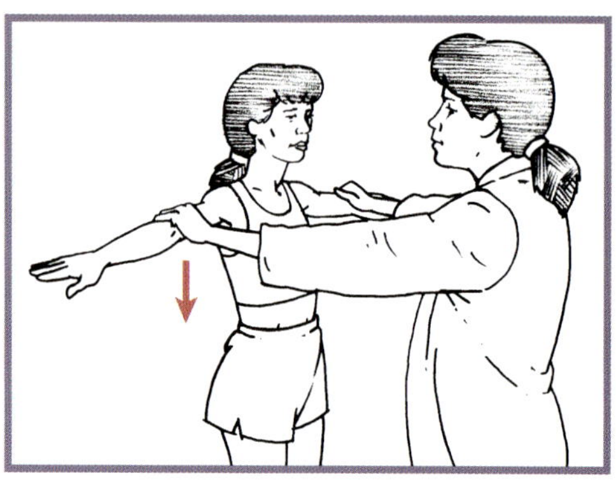

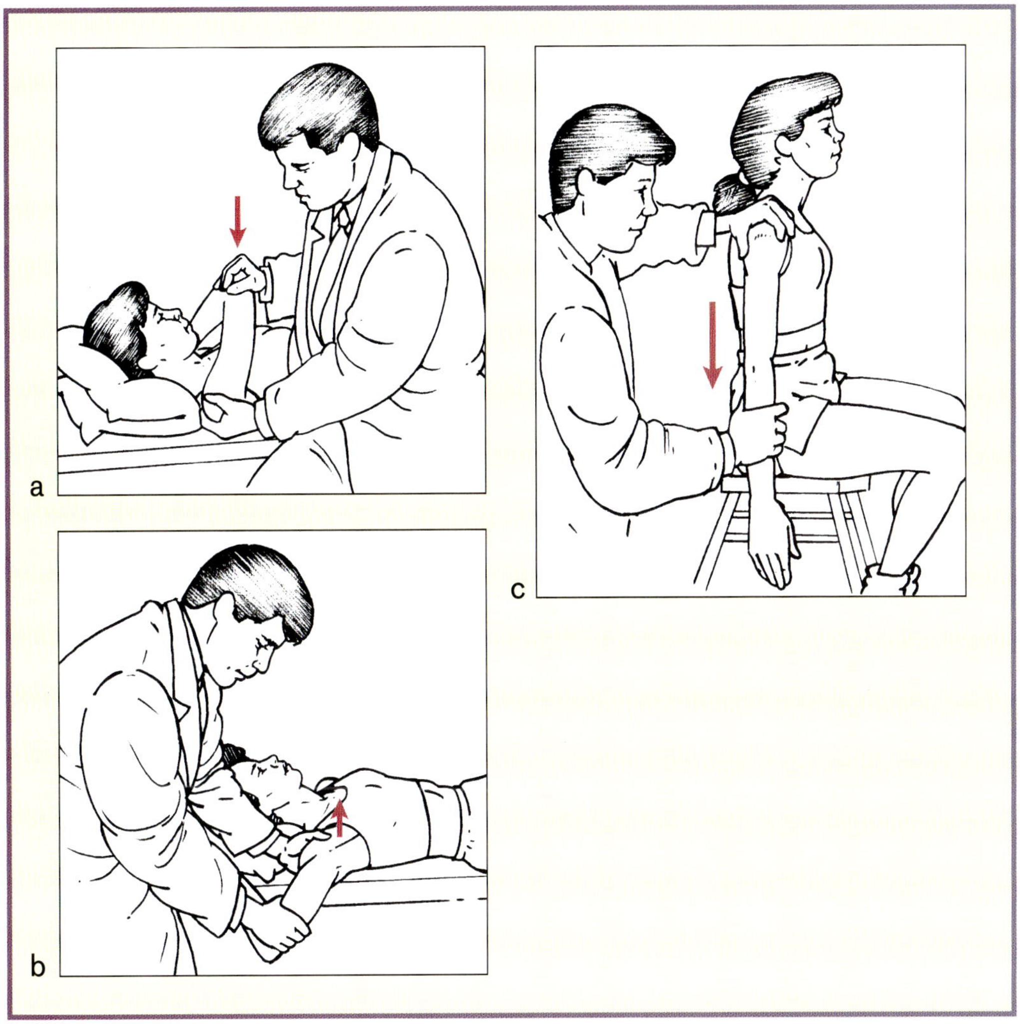

Figure 6.
Multidirectional instability can be gauged by assessing glenohumeral motion in several planes. Posterior instability of the shoulder is assessed in the supine athlete by positioning the arm perpendicular to the table with the elbow bent, then applying pressure along the long axis of the arm (a). The hand supporting the posterior shoulder palpates for excessive motion. To test anterior instability (b), the examiner abducts the athlete's shoulder, then lifts the humeral head anteriorly. In both tests, degree of motion, symmetry between the shoulders, and apprehension should be noted. With the athlete seated, inferior subluxation is confirmed by the presence of the sulcus sign—appearance of an indentation beneath the acromion with traction along the axis of the adducted arm (c).

flatfoot deformities should be noted. A supple flatfoot does not affect the athlete's performance but may be a risk factor for lower extremity overuse problems such as medial tibial stress syndrome or patellofemoral pain. If the flatfoot is supple, the plantar arch will increase when the athlete stands on his or her toes. Toe deformities, including bunions, contractures, and pressure points indicated by calluses, may become painful in athletic foot-wear.

Sport-specific examinations. Some sports medicine physicians advocate sport-specific physical examinations.[10,11] Such examinations focus on areas under particular stress (and therefore at higher risk for injury) in a given sport, and include strength, endurance, and flexibility testing in addition to a more general orthopedic examination. For example, for swimmers and baseball pitchers an examiner might measure shoulder internal and external rotation strength and endurance with isokinetic testing; for running and jumping athletes the examiner might test knee flexion, extension, and strength with isokinetic testing, and observe gait biomechanics on a treadmill. Although such precisely focused tests may reveal information that can improve performance and possibly

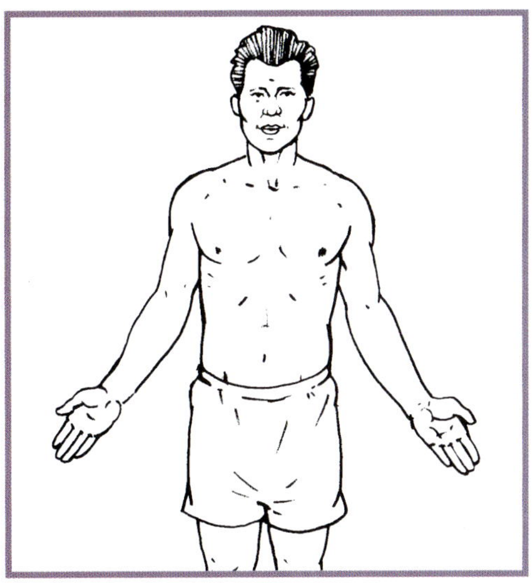

Figure 7.
The normal carrying angle of the elbow is at least 15° valgus with the athlete standing and the palms forward. An excessive valgus angle may indicate instability or a previous injury.

Figure 8.
Hip range of motion is evaluated with the athlete supine. As part of the examination, the hip and knee are flexed to 90°, and the hip joint is rotated. A rotation arc of at least 60° should be observed. Pain or restriction of motion relative to the opposite side warrants further evaluation.

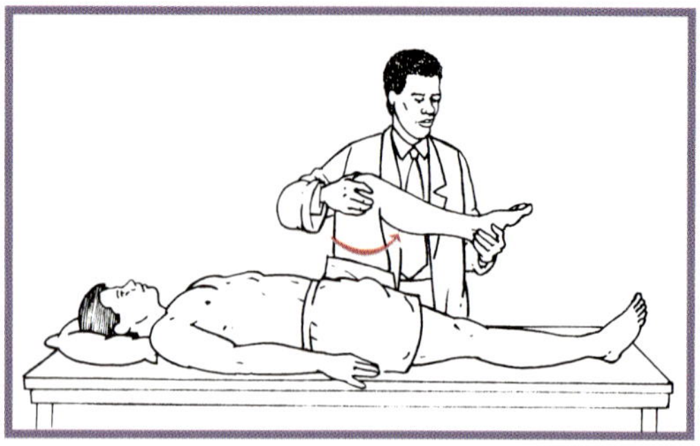

Figure 9.
Several tests are used to assess ligamentous instability of the knee. For each test, the degree of excursion and the quality of the endpoint are noted and compared with the opposite side. The Lachman test (a) is the most sensitive means to assess anterior cruciate ligament deficiencies. The patient's knee is flexed approximately 20°, and the muscles are relaxed. The examiner stabilizes the femur with one hand and grasps and pulls the tibia anteriorly with the other hand. The anterior and posterior drawer tests (b, c) can reveal anterior and posterior cruciate ligament insufficiency, respectively. With the supine patient's knee bent 90°, the examiner palpates the anteromedial tibial plateau for a tibia-femur step-off. Presence of a posterior tibial sag indicates laxity of the posterior cruciate ligament. Then the examiner sits on the patient's foot to stabilize it and grasps the proximal tibia. The hamstrings should be palpated to ensure they are relaxed. The examiner pulls the tibia anteriorly (anterior drawer test, b) and pushes it posteriorly (posterior drawer test, c) from the neutral position. With the anterior drawer test, lack of a firm endpoint and presence of excessive anterior tibial excursion suggest anterior cruciate ligament insufficiency. With the posterior drawer test, presence of excessive posterior tibial sag suggests posterior cruciate ligament insufficiency. Varus (d) and valgus (e) stress tests gauge instability of the medial and lateral collateral ligaments of the knee. The athlete's knee is extended over the edge of the examination table and flexed to approximately 20°. One of the examiner's hands stabilizes the knee at the joint line, and varus and valgus stresses are applied to the tibia. Comparison with the opposite limb is essential, given the normal range of variation in joint stability.

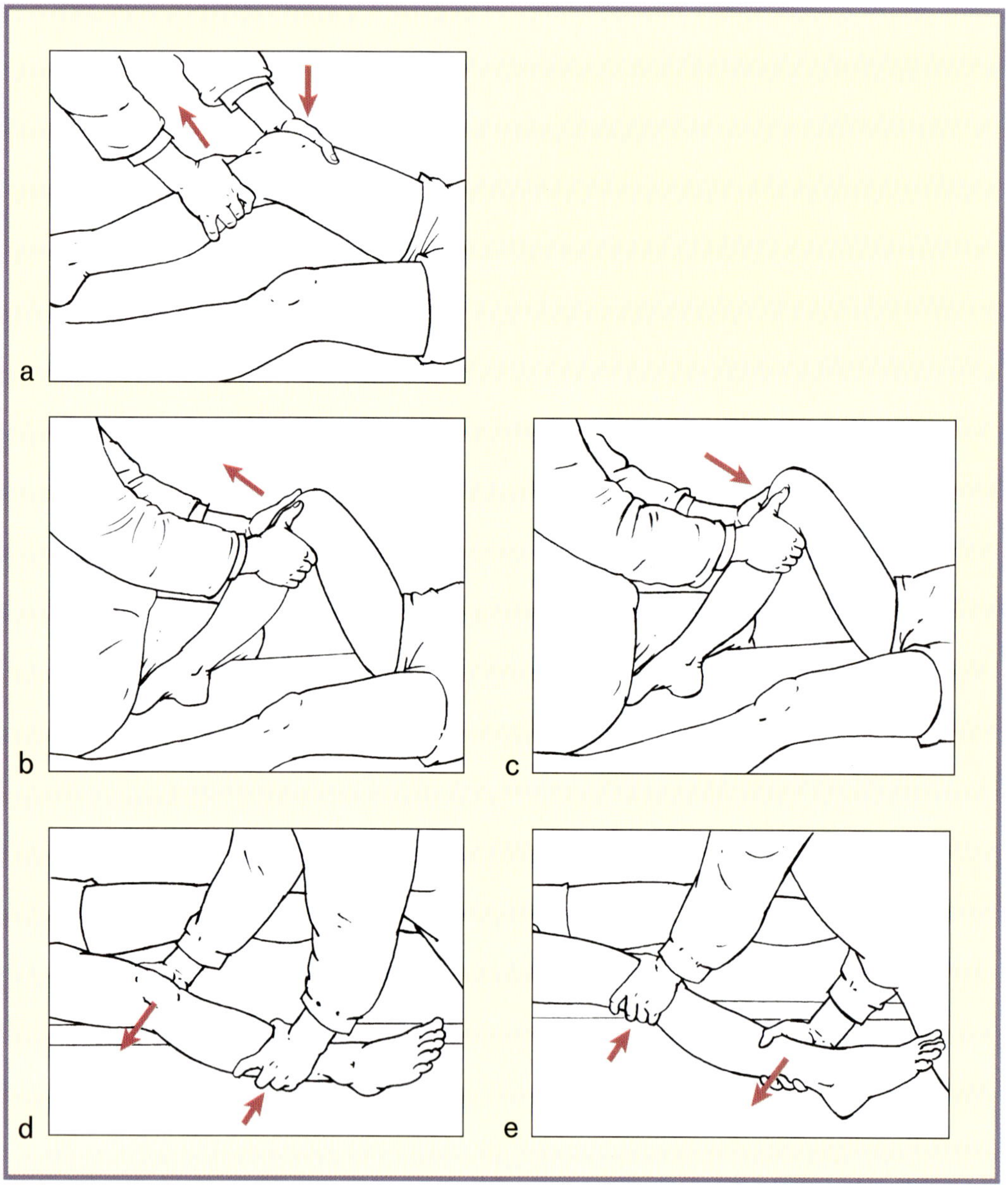

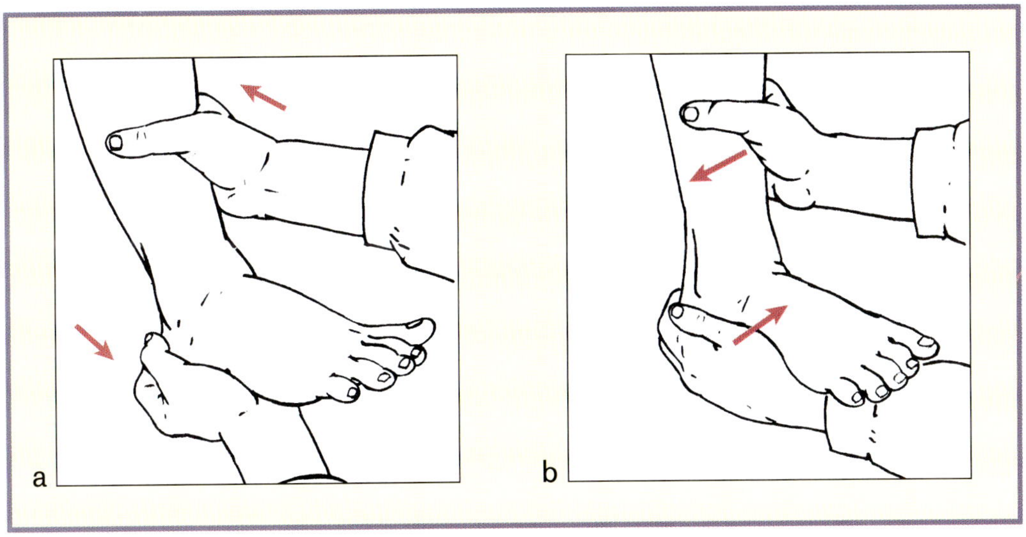

Figure 10.
Two stress tests are used to assess instability of the ankle ligaments. For the anterior drawer test (a), which demonstrates anterior subluxation, the examiner pulls the heel anteriorly while pushing posteriorly on the distal tibia. For the talar tilt test (b), the examiner inverts the ankle by pushing laterally on the medial tibia and medially on the calcaneus. Excessive motion, particularly relative to the opposite side, should trigger further evaluation.

prevent injury, these examinations are time-consuming and require more in-depth knowledge of individual sports than the joint-specific examination or the general screening examination. When time, resources, and expertise allow, however, such examinations can supplement or replace the general screening examination and/or the joint-specific examination.

NEUROLOGIC SYSTEM

In most cases, a normal musculoskeletal examination also implies normal motor neurologic function. However, additional neurologic testing may be required in certain situations. For example, in athletes with recurrent stingers/burners, an examination of the cervical spine and testing of upper extremity strength and deep tendon reflexes are appropriate. An athlete who has had multiple or severe concussions needs a detailed history of these concussions, as described on page 11, but may also require examination of cranial nerves and motor, cerebellar, and cognitive function. Referral for a more comprehensive neurologic evaluation is warranted if any impairment is noted or if limited time and/or clinical expertise of the examining physician does not allow adequate neurologic evaluation during the PPE.

Determining CLEARANCE

OVERVIEW

The most important and difficult decision in the PPE is determining clearance for sports participation. Clearance can be divided into three categories: (1) unrestricted clearance, (2) clearance after completion of further evaluation or rehabilitation, and (3) not cleared for certain types of sport or for all sports. Forms for recording clearance category are available on page 49.

If the athlete cannot play the sport of choice, the physician must consider alternatives that allow some form of participation. One study emphasized the importance of participation by pointing out that adolescents rank failure to make a team worse than death of a close friend, failure to pass a grade in school, and separation of parents.[51]

When an abnormality or condition is found that may limit an athlete's participation or predispose him or her to further injury, the physician must consider the following questions:

- Does the problem place the athlete at increased risk for injury?
- Is another participant at risk for injury because of the problem?
- Can the athlete safely participate with treatment (such as medication, rehabilitation, bracing, or padding)?
- Can limited participation be allowed while treatment is being completed?
- If clearance is denied only for certain sports or sport categories, in what activities can the athlete safely participate?

Clearance for a particular sport may be based on guidelines established by the 1994 American Academy of Pediatrics (AAP) Committee on Sports Medicine and Fitness (tables 5, 6, and 7)[52] or, for cardiovascular abnormalities, on the 26th Bethesda Conference guidelines.[46] These recommendations classify sports according to the degree of contact and dynamic and static strenuousness.

Contact categories (table 5) are based on the potential for injury from collision. High-impact contact/collision sports, such as football and ice hockey, have a higher risk of serious injury than noncontact sports, such as golf.

Distinctions based on strenuousness (table 6) are particularly relevant for athletes with cardiovascular or pulmonary disease. Static exercise causes a pressure load, whereas dynamic exercise causes a volume load on the left ventricle.[53]

The AAP has established participation guidelines (table 7) that may be used in deciding to clear an athlete for a particular sport. The physician's judgment is essential in applying these recommendations to a specific patient,[52] and alternative activities or treatment should be suggested when possible.

In the station-based evaluation, clearance should be determined at the last station. It is best performed by a physician who is familiar with the demands of the activities; the limitations that result from various problems; and the AAP, Bethesda, and similar relevant recommendations. The physician may also decide on follow-up and fur-

TABLE 5.

Classification of Sports by Contact

Contact/Collision	Limited Contact	Noncontact
Basketball	Baseball	Archery
Boxing*	Bicycling	Badminton
Diving	Cheerleading	Body building
Field hockey	Canoeing/Kayaking (white water)	Canoeing/Kayaking (flat water)
Football	Fencing	Crew/Rowing
Flag	Field	Curling
Tackle	High jump	Dancing
Ice hockey	Pole vault	Field
Lacrosse	Floor hockey	Discus
Martial arts	Gymnastics	Javelin
Rodeo	Handball	Shot put
Rugby	Horseback riding	Golf
Ski jumping	Racquetball	Orienteering
Soccer	Skating	Power lifting
Team handball	Ice	Race walking
Water polo	In-line	Riflery
Wrestling	Roller	Rope jumping
	Skiing	Running
	Cross-country	Sailing
	Downhill	Scuba diving
	Water	Strength training
	Softball	Swimming
	Squash	Table tennis
	Ultimate Frisbee	Tennis
	Volleyball	Track
	Windsurfing/Surfing	Weight lifting

**Participation not recommended by the AAP. The AAFP, AMSSM, AOASM, and AOSSM have no stand against boxing.*

Reprinted with permission from American Academy of Pediatrics Committee on Sports Medicine and Fitness: Medical conditions affecting sports participation. Pediatrics 1994;94(5):757-760

ther work-up for a specific problem. In the office setting, individual physicians should refer to the relevant recommendations as needed.

No matter which type of evaluation is done—private office or station screening—it is extremely important to ensure complete understanding by the athletes, parents, coaches, and, when necessary, school administrators, of any restrictions, necessary work-up and treatment, and any alternative activities in which the athlete may participate. To respect confidentiality, however, the physician involved in restricting an athlete should obtain authorization from the athlete and parent(s) or guardian(s) if the athlete is a minor prior to releasing information to coaches and school administrators.

Using a clearance form separate from the history and physical examination form, such as that on page 49, is suggested as a means of providing the parent(s) and school with a copy of clearance decisions and follow-up recommendations while protecting the confidentiality of the athlete's history and physical findings. Alternatively, this form may be used just for athletes who are not fully cleared.

Occasionally, an athlete will wish to participate despite medical recommendations to the contrary. In such cases, it is critical that the athlete, his or her parent(s) or guardian(s), the coach, and school or program administrators all understand the degree of risk in participation and the potential long-term consequences of participation. (See page 43 for a discussion of participation rights and exculpatory waivers.)

TABLE 6.

Classification of Sports by Strenuousness

High-to-Moderate Intensity

High-to-Moderate Dynamic and Static Demands	High-to-Moderate Dynamic and Low Static Demands	High-to-Moderate Static and Low Dynamic Demands
Boxing*	Badminton	Archery
Crew/Rowing	Baseball	Auto racing
Cross-country skiing	Basketball	Diving
Cycling	Field hockey	Equestrian
Downhill skiing	Lacrosse	Field events (jumping)
Fencing	Orienteering	Field events (throwing)
Football	Ping-pong	Gymnastics
Ice Hockey	Race walking	Karate or judo
Rugby	Racquetball	Motorcycling
Running (sprint)	Soccer	Rodeoing
Speed skating	Squash	Sailing
Water polo	Swimming	Ski jumping
Wrestling	Tennis	Water skiing
	Volleyball	Weight lifting

Low Intensity

Low Dynamic and Low Static Demands
Bowling
Cricket
Curling
Golf
Riflery

**Participation not recommended by the AAP. The AAFP, AMSSM, AOASM, and AOSSM have no stand against boxing.*

Reprinted with permission from American Academy of Pediatrics Committee on Sports Medicine and Fitness: Medical conditions affecting sports participation. Pediatrics 1994;94(5):757-760

ALCOHOL AND DRUG USE

Competitors need to be aware of the names and dosages of the drugs and supplements they are taking and the policies that affect them. Regulations vary by organization; appropriately trained sports medicine providers should be familiar with guidelines relevant to their institution. The NCAA Sports Medicine Handbook supplies information on NCAA regulations, and can be ordered through the association's circulation department (913/339-1906). Information on USOC regulations may be obtained by writing to: Drug Control Administration, United States Olympic Committee, 1 Olympic Plaza, Colorado Springs, CO 80909.

ACUTE ILLNESS

Because the PPE is performed in advance of the sports season, denial of participation because of an acute illness does not generally occur. When it is an issue, clearance should be based on individual assessment. Factors to consider include the risk of the illness worsening as a result of participation and the potential for spreading the disease to others. AAP guidelines disallow participation during febrile illness and with all but mild diarrhea; many clinicians individualize the decision on the basis of clinical findings such as constitutional symptoms. Limiting activity in patients with fever and/or diarrhea is important in minimizing the risk of complications secondary to dehydration, thermoregulatory problems, and viral infection (especially myocarditis, although this is rare).

TABLE 7.

Medical Conditions and Sports Participation

This table is designed to be understood by medical and nonmedical personnel. In the "Explanation" section below, "needs evaluation" means that a physician with appropriate knowledge and experience should assess the safety of a given sport for an athlete with the listed medical condition. Unless otherwise noted, this is because of the variability of the severity of the disease or of the risk of injury among the specific sports, or both.

Condition	May Participate
Atlantoaxial instability* (instability of the joint between cervical vertebrae 1 and 2) Explanation: Athlete needs evaluation to assess risk of spinal cord injury during sports participation.	**Qualified Yes**
Bleeding disorder* Explanation: Athlete needs evaluation.	**Qualified Yes**
Cardiovascular diseases	
Carditis (inflammation of the heart) Explanation: Carditis may result in sudden death with exertion.	**No**
Hypertension (high blood pressure) Explanation: Those with significant essential (unexplained) hypertension should avoid weight and power lifting, body building, and strength training. Those with secondary hypertension (hypertension caused by a previously identified disease), or severe essential hypertension, need evaluation.†	**Qualified Yes**
Congenital heart disease (structural heart defects present at birth) Explanation: Those with mild forms may participate fully; those with moderate or severe forms, or who have undergone surgery, need evaluation.‡	**Qualified Yes**
Dysrhythmia (irregular heart rhythm) Explanation: Athlete needs evaluation because some types require therapy or make certain sports dangerous, or both.	**Qualified Yes**
Mitral valve prolapse (abnormal heart valve) Explanation: Those with symptoms (chest pain, symptoms of possible dysrhythmia) or evidence of mitral regurgitation (leaking) on physical examination need evaluation. All others may participate fully.	**Qualified Yes**
Heart murmur Explanation: If the murmur is innocent (does not indicate heart disease), full participation is permitted. Otherwise, the athlete needs evaluation (see "Congenital heart disease" and "Mitral valve prolapse" above).	**Qualified Yes**
Cerebral Palsy* Explanation: Athlete needs evaluation.	**Qualified Yes**
Diabetes mellitus*§ Explanation: All sports can be played with proper attention to diet, hydration, and insulin therapy. Particular attention is needed for activities that last 30 minutes or more.	**Yes**
Diarrhea¶ Explanation: Unless disease is mild, no participation is permitted, because diarrhea may increase the risk of dehydration and heat illness. See "Fever" below.	**Qualified No**
Eating disorders	
Anorexia nervosa, Bulimia nervosa Explanation: These patients need both medical and psychiatric assessment before participation.	**Qualified Yes**
Eyes	
Functionally one-eyed athlete, loss of an eye, detached retina, previous eye surgery or serious eye injury Explanation: A functionally one-eyed athlete has a best corrected visual acuity of <20/40 in the worse eye. These athletes would suffer significant disability if the better eye was seriously injured as would those with loss of an eye. Some athletes who have previously undergone eye surgery or had a serious eye injury may have an increased risk of injury because of weakened eye tissue. Availability of eye guards approved by the American Society for Testing Materials (ASTM) and other protective equipment may allow participation in most sports, but this must be judged on an individual basis.	**Qualified Yes**
Fever¶ Explanation: Fever can increase cardiopulmonary effort, reduce maximum exercise capacity, make heat illness more likely, and increase orthostatic hypotension during exercise. Fever may rarely accompany myocarditis or other infections that may make exercise dangerous.	**No**
Heat illness, history of Explanation: Because of the increased likelihood of recurrence, the athlete needs individual assessment to determine the presence of predisposing conditions and to arrange a prevention strategy.	**Qualified Yes**
HIV infection¶ Explanation: Because of the apparent minimal risk to others, all sports may be played that the state of health allows. In all athletes, skin lesions should be properly covered, and athletic personnel should use universal precautions when handling blood or body fluids with visible blood.	**Yes**

Condition	May Participate
Kidney: absence of one Explanation: Athlete needs individual assessment for contact/collision and limited contact sports.	Qualified Yes
Liver, enlarged Explanation: If the liver is acutely enlarged, participation should be avoided because of risk of rupture. If the liver is chronically enlarged, individual assessment is needed before contact/collision or limited contact sports are played.	Qualified Yes
Malignancy* Explanation: Athlete needs individual assessment.	Qualified Yes
Musculoskeletal disorders Explanation: Athlete needs individual assessment.	Qualified Yes
Neurologic	
History of serious head or spine trauma, severe or repeated concussions, or craniotomy Explanation: Athlete needs individual assessment for contact/collision or limited contact sports, and also for noncontact sports if there are deficits in judgment or cognition. Recent research supports a conservative approach to management of concussion.	Qualified Yes
Convulsive disorder, well controlled Explanation: Risk of convulsion during participation is minimal.	Yes
Convulsive disorder, poorly controlled Explanation: Athlete needs individual assessment for contact/collision or limited contact sports. Avoid the following noncontact sports: archery, riflery, swimming, weight or power lifting, strength training, or sports involving heights. In these sports, occurrence of a convulsion may be a risk to self or others.	Qualified Yes
Obesity Explanation: Because of the risk of heat illness, obese persons need careful acclimatization and hydration.	Qualified Yes
Organ transplant recipient* Explanation: Athlete needs individual assessment.	Qualified Yes
Ovary: absence of one Explanation: Risk of severe injury to the remaining ovary is minimal.	Yes
Respiratory	
Pulmonary compromise including cystic fibrosis* Explanation: Athlete needs individual assessment, but generally all sports may be played if oxygenation remains satisfactory during a graded exercise test. Patients with cystic fibrosis need acclimatization and good hydration to reduce the risk of heat illness.	Qualified Yes
Asthma Explanation: With proper medication and education, only athletes with the most severe asthma will have to modify their participation.	Yes
Acute upper respiratory infection Explanation: Upper respiratory obstruction may affect pulmonary function. Athlete needs individual assessment for all but mild disease. See "Fever" above.	Qualified Yes
Sickle cell disease Explanation: Athlete needs individual assessment. In general, if status of the illness permits, all but high-exertion, contact/collision sports may be played. Overheating, dehydration, and chilling must be avoided.	Qualified Yes
Sickle cell trait Explanation: It is unlikely that individuals with sickle cell trait (AS) have an increased risk of sudden death or other medical problems during athletic participation except under the most extreme conditions of heat, humidity, and possibly increased altitude. These individuals, like all athletes, should be carefully conditioned, acclimatized, and hydrated to reduce any possible risk.	Yes
Skin: boils, herpes simplex, impetigo, scabies, molluscum contagiosum Explanation: While the patient is contagious, participation in gymnastics with mats, martial arts, wrestling, or other contact/collision or limited contact sports is not allowed. Herpes simplex virus probably is not transmitted via mats.	Qualified Yes
Spleen, enlarged¶ Explanation: Patients with acutely enlarged spleens should avoid all sports because of risk of rupture. Those with chronically enlarged spleens need individual assessment before playing contact/collision or limited contact sports.	Qualified Yes
Testicle: absent or undescended Explanation: Certain sports may require a protective cup.	Yes

** Not discussed in text of the monograph. † See table 4. ‡ Mild, moderate, and severe congenital heart disease are defined in 26th Bethesda Conference: Recommendations for determining eligibility for competition in athletes with cardiovascular abnormalities. January 6-7, 1994. Med Sci Sports Exerc 1994;26(10 suppl):S246-253*

§ Well controlled. ¶ AAP recommendation as indicated; see text for qualifications by other commentators.

Reprinted with permission from: American Academy of Pediatrics Committee on Sports Medicine and Fitness: Medical conditions affecting sports participation. Pediatrics 1994;94(5):757-760

BLOOD-BORNE PATHOGENS

The blood-borne pathogens of greatest concern in sports at present are HIV and the hepatitis B, C, and D viruses. HIV is transmitted through sexual contact, parenteral exposure to blood and blood products, contamination of open wounds or mucous membranes with infected blood, and perinatal spread from an infected mother to her baby. HIV is also present in tears, sweat, urine, sputum, vomitus, saliva, and respiratory droplets, but only blood is recognized as a threat in the athletic setting. HIV transmission during sports has only been suspected in one case in an Italian soccer player in 1990.[54] However, this report was poorly documented and is not universally accepted as a transmission related to sport. Transmission of HIV has never been shown to occur in the NFL; the risk of transmission can be estimated to be less than one transmission per one million games.[55]

The hepatitis B, C, and D viruses (HBV, HCV, and HDV) are spread in the same manner as HIV (sexually, parenterally, and perinatally). HBV-infected blood is known to contain 100 million infectious doses of the virus per milliliter,[56] whereas HIV is reported to contain only a few hundred to a few thousand particles per milliliter.[57] Despite this difference, only one case of HBV transmission in sport has been reported, involving high school sumo wrestlers in Japan in 1982.[58] HCV was recognized as a cause of non-A, non-B hepatitis in 1989; it accounts for 20% to 50% of all cases of hepatitis in the United States.[59] HDV depends on the presence of HBV for expression, and often causes progressive liver disease and fulminant hepatitis. Neither HCV nor HDV has been shown to have an increased incidence as a result of sports participation.

Participation by the HIV-infected athlete is a complex issue. First and foremost, the health status of the individual must be considered. HIV infection, though ultimately and uniformly fatal, often allows an asymptomatic period of good health during which prophylactic treatment should be instituted according to current medical practice. Positive HIV status in an asymptomatic individual does not by itself mandate discontinuation of athletic participation.[32] Moderate-intensity exercise has been shown to be beneficial to asymptomatic HIV-positive patients.[60] Proper care by a physician who understands the demands of the individual sport is paramount. The type of athletic activity, the athlete's current health status, health risks of participation, intensity of training, and risk of transmission to others all need to be considered. Confidentiality of the health status of the individual must also be maintained. Athletes must be counseled on the legal requirement of physicians to report positive HIV cases.

Infection with HBV, HCV, or HDV should be viewed as any other viral infection. Clinical symptoms of fatigue, fever, malaise, anorexia, and abdominal pain should be evaluated in relation to the demands of athletic participation. Asymptomatic individuals may participate in sport under the guidance and monitoring of a knowledgeable physician.

CARDIOVASCULAR ABNORMALITIES

Clearance guidelines for cardiovascular conditions in young athletes have been established by considering which conditions may be exacerbated by physical activity and which predispose an athlete to sudden cardiac death during activity. The practical guidelines established by the 26th Bethesda Conference[46] cover the major cardiac abnormalities seen in athletes, including hypertension, arrhythmias, congenital heart disease, acquired valvular disease, ischemic heart disease, and the cardiomyopathies. It is recommended that any physician who clears athletes for participation do so in accordance with this reference. If any doubts remain about the cardiovascular condition after thorough evaluation by the athlete's personal physician, full evaluation and clearance should be performed by a cardiologist.

Summaries of the Bethesda guidelines for several common cardiac conditions follow:

Hypertension. Athletes who have mild-to-moderate hypertension and no evidence of end-organ damage may compete in all categories of sports but should be treated and have regular monitoring of their blood pressure. Those who have severe hypertension should not be allowed to compete in any sport until their hypertension is evaluated and treated, at which time eligibility for participation can be reevaluated. Therefore, unless hypertension first noted at the PPE is severe, the athlete may be cleared for competition while the condition is evaluated. If end-organ damage is suspected, further evaluation is indicated.

Benign functional murmurs. These are commonly found during the PPE but do not preclude participation in sports (see also pages 10, 18).

Mitral valve prolapse. This condition should not restrict an athlete from participation in high-intensity competitive sports unless accompanied by one of the following: (1) history of syncope due to arrhythmia, (2) family history of sudden death attributed to mitral valve prolapse, (3) prior embolic event, (4) arrhythmia (eg, supraventricular arrhythmias) worsened by exercise, or (5) moderate-to-marked mitral regurgitation. If any of these criteria apply, participation in low-intensity sports may be considered on an individual basis.

Hypertrophic cardiomyopathy. Athletes with an unequivocal diagnosis of HCM, the most common cause of sudden death in young athletes,[34] should not be allowed to participate in competitive sports, with the possible exception of low-intensity sports as defined by the 26th Bethesda conference.[61] Though some nationally known athletes have been allowed to play in dynamic sports, recommendations for risk stratification in HCM cannot be made in athletes younger than 30 years. Evaluation and recommendations should be made on an individual basis.

Arrhythmias. Although a discussion of arrhythmias is beyond the scope of this monograph, recommendations for clearance of athletes are covered in the 26th Bethesda Conference guidelines.[46]

DERMATOLOGIC DISORDERS

The presence of an infectious dermatologic condition, such as herpes simplex, scabies, louse infestation, molluscum contagiosum, impetigo, or furuncles/carbuncles, precludes participation in some contact/collision sports. Play may be resumed when the condition has resolved or is no longer contagious. Denying clearance is especially important in sports in which mats are used, such as wrestling, gymnastics, and martial arts, and in sports in which equipment such as baseball helmets is shared.

DISORDERED EATING AND THE FEMALE ATHLETE TRIAD

When disordered eating or the female athlete triad (interrelated disordered eating, amenorrhea, and osteopenia) is suspected, evaluation and treatment, using a multidisciplinary approach, is warranted. Athletes may be reluctant to undergo treatment, but their cooperation is imperative. It must be stressed with coaches and athletes that disordered eating patterns may impair athletic performance and predispose the athlete to recurrent injury, particularly stress fractures. Recovery is often a lengthy process.

Athletic participation should be restricted when there is evidence of compromised performance or when disordered eating or the female athlete triad has threatened the athlete's health in such a way that continued participation could cause injury.[62]

EYE DISORDERS

The potential for loss of vision because of injury is always a concern in sports, but is particularly acute for athletes whose vision is already impaired in one eye. For such athletes, loss of the better eye may result in a significant change in lifestyle.[64] For instance, several states will not issue a driver's license if the best corrected vision is less than 20/40. Consequently, athletes with best corrected vision in one eye of less than 20/40 should be considered functionally one-eyed.

Sports in which eye protection cannot be effectively worn are contraindicated for functionally one-eyed athletes (table 8). These athletes who participate in such sports as football, racquetball, baseball, or basketball, which involve a high risk of eye injury, may be individually evaluated and allowed to participate if they wear appropriate protective eyewear (table 8).

The athlete, his or her parent(s) or

TABLE 8.

Sports With High Risk of Eye Injury, With Appropriate Eye Protectors

Sport	Eye Protection*
Badminton	Sports goggles with polycarbonate lenses
Baseball	Polycarbonate face guard or other certified safe protection attached to helmet for batting and base running; sports goggles with polycarbonate lenses for fielding
Bicycling (LER)†	Sturdy street-wear frames with polycarbonate or CR-39 lenses
Boxing	None is available
Fencing	Full face cage
Field hockey (both sexes)	Goalie: full face mask; all others: sports goggles with polycarbonate lenses
Football	Polycarbonate shield on helmet
Full-contact martial arts	Not allowed
Handball‡	Sports goggles with polycarbonate lenses
Ice hockey	Helmet and full face protection
Lacrosse (male)	Helmet and full face protection required
Lacrosse (female)	Should at least wear sports goggles with polycarbonate lenses and have option to wear helmet and full face protection
Racquetball‡	Sports goggles with polycarbonate lenses
Soccer	Sports goggles with polycarbonate lenses
Softball	Polycarbonate face guard or other certified safe protection attached to helmet for batting and base running; sports goggles with polycarbonate lenses for fielding
Squash‡	Sports goggles with polycarbonate lenses
Street hockey	Sports goggles with polycarbonate lenses; goalie: full face cage
Swimming and pool sports	Swim goggles recommended
Tennis: doubles	Sports goggles with polycarbonate lenses
Tennis: singles	Sturdy street-wear frames with polycarbonate lenses
Track and field (LER)†	Sturdy street-wear frames with polycarbonate or CR-39 lenses
Water polo	Swim goggles with polycarbonate lenses
Wrestling	None is available

** For sports in which a face mask or helmet with eye protection is worn, functionally one-eyed athletes, and those with previous eye trauma or surgery for whom their ophthalmologists recommend eye protection, must also wear sports goggles with polycarbonate lenses to ensure protection.*

† LER = Low Eye Risk

‡ Goggles without lenses are not effective.

§ A street hockey ball can penetrate into a molded goalie mask and injure an eye.

Used by permission. American Academy of Pediatrics, American Academy of Ophthalmology: Protective eyewear for young athletes. Pediatrics, August 1996. To be published.

guardian(s), the coach, and school administrators, if necessary, must understand what the serious long-term consequences of injury to the better eye would be, the level of protection available for the better eye, and the degree of risk of injury—with and without protection—to the better eye. Treatments for injuries that can typically occur in the desired activity should also be discussed.

If, after this discussion, the athlete still wishes to participate in a given sport, he or she must wear appropriate protective eyewear during participation (see also pages 29, 43).

If the athlete has had previous significant eye injury or has had eye surgery, referral to an ophthalmologist is recommended for complete evaluation and clearance. If an athlete has sustained a detached retina, consultation with an ophthalmologist should be obtained before allowing the athlete to return to competition.

GYNECOLOGIC DISORDERS, PREGNANCY

Because ovarian injury is so unlikely in sports, no restrictions are necessary for female athletes with only one ovary. Athletes with menstrual disorders usually may be cleared while undergoing further evaluation (see also page 16). However, if pregnancy is suspected, clearance for contact/collision or strenuous sports participation should be withheld pending either a negative pregnancy test or clearance by the clinician who is following the pregnancy. Although the examiner may refer an athlete for a Pap smear, it is not usually necessary to delay clearance in such cases.

HEAT ILLNESS, RECURRENT

Because of the increased likelihood of recurrence, the athlete with prior heat illness needs individual assessment to determine the presence of predisposing conditions and to arrange a prevention strategy. Recurrent heat illness may be due to a medical condition, such as obesity or febrile illness; medications, such as antihistamines, antidepressants, or psychomotor stimulants; dehydration; or insufficient acclimatization. All of these may be addressed with a thorough discussion of prevention, and clearance need not be denied. However, if the athlete has a documented history of heatstroke or heat-related rhabdomyolysis, further investigation of the previous diagnostic work-up is warranted. Clearance for these athletes may be restricted to participation under temperate conditions.

HEPATOMEGALY AND SPLENOMEGALY

Organomegaly is a cause of concern if there is increased risk of damage to the organ or malfunction of a vital organ. The underlying etiology must also be determined.

Acute hepatomegaly may signal the presence of infection (eg, hepatitis, infectious mononucleosis) or malignant disease (eg, hepatocellular carcinoma, lymphoma). A liver that is enlarged beyond the bony protection of the rib cage is at risk for injury. Even though the incidence of hepatic rupture among patients with acute hepatomegaly is low, participation in all sports should be avoided. Full activity may be resumed after resolution of hepatomegaly.

An athlete who has acute splenomegaly should not participate in sports. This recommendation is based on reports of spleen rupture in individuals engaged in nonstrenuous activities, even a simple Valsalva's maneuver.

For individuals with chronic hepatomegaly/splenomegaly, participation in sports should be assessed individually and decisions based on the degree of enlargement and the associated disease state.

INGUINAL HERNIA

In the past, athletes with an inguinal hernia were removed from all but noncontact activities. However, it is now agreed that such athletes can participate in any activity. A symptomatic inguinal hernia may limit an athlete's ability to participate and may be affected by activity. The symptomatic cases invariably require treatment at some time and should be evaluated individually. It may be wise to have an athlete with an inguinal hernia consult a general surgeon in case symptoms requiring elective or emergency surgery arise.

KIDNEY ABNORMALITIES

Because of the potential for kidney injuries ranging from contusion to complete rupture, special consideration should be given when determining clearance for an athlete who has a single functioning kidney. Some, but not all, experts believe that if the kidney is pelvic, iliac, multicystic, or shows evidence of hydronephrosis or ureteropelvic junction abnormalities, the athlete should not participate in contact/collision sports. The consequences of the loss of a single functioning kidney (transplantation or dialysis) may be severe enough to warrant disqualification from these sports, even though the risk is small. Evaluation by an specialist is recommended. If the single kidney is normal, the athlete may participate but should be advised as to the risk involved.

If the athlete chooses to play in a sport that may place a solitary kidney at increased risk for damage, a full explanation should be given to the athlete, his or her parent(s) or guardian(s), and the coaches. The explanation should include available protection, potential serious long-term consequences, and treatment of injuries if they occur (see also pages 29, 43).

MUSCULOSKELETAL DISORDERS

Determining clearance for athletes who have musculoskeletal injuries or disorders requires assessing both short- and long-term risks and benefits, considering carefully the general questions on page 29. Clearance for participation must be based on the degree and type of injury, the ability of the injured athlete to compete safely, and the requirements of a given sport. Participation may be possible in activities not directly affecting the injured part (eg, a wrist sprain might keep a gymnast but not a runner out of play). This latitude offers the athlete the opportunity to compete or maintain conditioning while not aggravating the injury.

Protective padding, taping, or bracing may be designed to provide the athlete a safe means to compete. Consultation with a sports medicine specialist may be necessary before such devices are prescribed.

Referral to an appropriate consultant is warranted when the examiner is uncertain of clearance guidelines. In any case, physicians involved with the treatment of an injury present at the time of the PPE should be included in the clearance decision. Reevaluation is required after rehabilitation.

Review of every musculoskeletal problem is beyond the scope of this monograph, but selected problems deserve mention:

Sprains, subluxations, and dislocations. Before clearance is given, sprains, subluxations, and dislocations should be examined and the following ruled out:

- Effusion, swelling, or other signs of inflammation;
- Decreased range of motion of the affected joint;
- Strength less than 85% to 90% of the uninjured side or insufficient for the desired activity;
- Ligamentous instability of the affected joint; and
- Loss or alteration of functional ability (ie, inability to complete pain-free functional activity at 100% effort). For example, on completion of rehabilitation for a lateral ankle sprain in a football defensive back this could be assessed with backpedalling and side-to-side motion.

Treatment should be instituted if any of these tests is abnormal. Multidirectional or unidirectional instability of the shoulder needs further evaluation and possible rehabilitation before clearance is given. Referral, if necessary, to a physician familiar with sports requirements and injury assessment is recommended. The decision for clearance is based on the examiner's clinical judgment and may be withheld until further evaluation and completion of prescribed treatment or rehabilitation. Further evaluation is warranted if uncertainty about clearance persists.

Strains or muscle contusions. Before clearance is given, strains or muscle contusions should be examined and the following ruled out:

- Decreased range of motion of joints controlled by the muscle;
- Strength less than 85% to 90% of the uninjured side or insufficient for the desired activity; and
- Loss or alteration of functional ability.

Treatment and clearance decisions parallel those for sprains, subluxations, and dislocations (above).

Overuse injuries. Overuse or overload injuries are caused by recurrent microtrauma, resulting initially in pain and inflammation and sometimes leading to tissue failure and potential disability. Examples of overuse injuries include stress fractures, Achilles tendinitis, medial and lateral epicondylitis, plantar fasciitis, patellofemoral pain syndrome, rotator cuff tendinitis, and impingement syndrome. Treatment and clearance decisions are based on criteria similar to those for acute sprains or strains.

Fractures. Clearance of an athlete with a fracture should be determined by the treating physician. The location, type, risk of reinjury or irreparable damage, and the effect of treatment should be considered. The possibility of protecting the fracture during participation with a playing cast or splint should be considered if the risk of worsening the injury is negligible. Also, in making clearance decisions, the physician should be aware of specific rules relevant to their athletes regarding use of unpadded hard materials on the extremities. Referral to a sports medicine specialist is warranted when the examiner's familiarity with a protective device or injury is incomplete.

Developmental conditions. Any history or physical findings of spinal deformity (eg, scoliosis, spondylolysis, spondylolisthesis) requires a more thorough evaluation than is generally provided in the PPE. Follow-up with the athlete's primary care physician or sports medicine specialist is recommended should questions arise. Spondylolysis and spondylolisthesis should be evaluated individually on the basis of symptoms, physical limitations, and x-ray findings. Because of the risk of progressive slippage, spondylolisthesis may require follow-up x-rays. Generally, athletes with spinal deformities need not be excluded from play. However, they should be educated about limiting activities that may cause progression of the deformity (eg, heavy axial loading activities, such as squatting with weights or overhead weight lifting).

Clearing athletes with apophysitis of the tibial tubercle (Osgood-Schlatter disease), calcaneus (Sever's disease), ilium, or ischium depends on the same criteria as for overuse injuries and acute strains.

If there are any questions concerning clearance, sports medicine consultation is suggested.

NEUROLOGIC DISORDERS

Because it is rare for an athlete to present for a PPE with an acute neurologic problem, the screening physician will more likely be determining clearance for athletes with a history of such problems as head or brain injury, burners/stingers, or convulsive disorders.

Concussion. The most common serious head injury in contact/collision sports is the cerebral concussion, with an estimated 250,000 such injuries occurring annually in football alone.[64] Although the definition of concussion is not universally agreed upon, a generally accepted and clinically useful definition is that a concussion is a traumatically induced alteration in mental status.[65] Likewise, disagreement persists among sports medicine specialists about classification of concussion severity and management and clearance guidelines.[66,67]

Furthermore, the cumulative effect of concussions is currently unknown.[68,69]

Despite the lack of scientific research to assist physicians in determining clearance for athletes who have a history of concussion, familiarity with the commonly referenced classification and management guidelines[64,65,70-72] is recommended. Individual assessment and clinical judgment should prevail, but, generally, athletes with a history of concussion who have been asymptomatic for an extended period and show no residual neurologic deficits are allowed to participate in all sports. If, however, an athlete presents for a PPE with a recent history of concussion and symptoms of postconcussion syndrome (eg, cognitive and/or memory impairment, irritability, headache, depression, anxiety, fatigue, or dizziness),[73] the examining physician should restrict the athlete from contact/collision sports until further evaluation by a neurologist or other clinician with expertise in this area.

One reason for caution in giving clearance after a concussion is the potential for a rare but catastrophic entity termed *second impact syndrome*. The syndrome results from a minor head injury in an individual recovering from previous trauma such as a mild concussion. It is thought that the cumulative damage disrupts the brain's blood autoregulation, with resultant brain swelling and increased intracranial pressure causing high morbidity and mortality.[65,74,75]

Burners/stingers and transient quadriparesis. Athletes who have had burners/stingers (nerve root or brachial plexus injury) may be cleared for all sports if they are asymptomatic and their physical examination is normal. Recurrent burners/stingers may require evaluation with cervical spine radiographs to rule out a predisposing condition such as cervical spine instability or degenerative changes. Athletes with a history of cervical spinal cord neurapraxia with transient quadriplegia should be evaluated fully, and referral to a spine specialist is suggested. Transient quadriplegia has been regarded as a contraindication to contact/collision sports when objective structural problems are noted. These patients should be treated on a case-by-case basis.[76-78]

Convulsive disorder. Because the literature is scarce regarding seizure disorders and risk of participation in sports, participation in potentially dangerous sports must be carefully considered. Current AAP guidelines (table 7) clear athletes who have a well-controlled convulsive disorder for participation in conventional school-sponsored sports. However, if a sport entails high risk (eg, skiing, gymnastics on high apparatus, high diving) and concern persists, consultation with or referral to a neurologist may be warranted.

When athletes have poorly controlled seizures, clearance should be deferred for contact/collision, limited contact, and potentially hazardous noncontact sports, such as archery, riflery, swimming, weight or power lifting, strength training, or sports involving heights. In the interim, while medications are adjusted and seizures are coming under control, athletes may participate in noncontact sports that do not involve risk to themselves or others. Consultation with a neurologist is recommended if there are further concerns or difficulties with seizure control. If athletic activity precipitates an athlete's seizures, clearance should be denied and the athlete referred as necessary.

PULMONARY DISORDERS

The most prevalent—although often overlooked—pulmonary problem in the PPE is EIA. There is no reason to withhold an athlete with asthma from participation in sports, although appropriate treatment is necessary to ensure optimal performance. A current diagnostic and therapeutic approach is to initiate a therapeutic trial of medication in athletes with a suspicious history, followed by an exercise test with pulmonary function monitoring for those in whom the trial does not improve function. Some physicians also use a methacholine challenge in diagnosing EIA. The medication most often used is a beta-agonist taken by inhalation; the clinician must ensure that the athlete is using the inhaler correctly.

Although it is infrequently detected during the PPE, severe pulmonary insufficiency (FEV_1 less than 50%), such as in pulmonary hypertension, cor pulmonale, or cystic fibrosis, requires referral for exercise stress testing and management.

SICKLE CELL TRAIT/DISEASE

In the United States, about 8% of blacks and approximately 0.8% of nonblacks have sickle cell trait. In this heterozygous condition, less than 50% of the hemoglobin is abnormal and there generally is no associated anemia. No evidence suggests any impaired exercise performance or increased risk of sudden death during normal conditions, and restricting these patients from activity under normal conditions is therefore unnecessary.[79] Under the most extreme conditions of heat, humidity, and possibly increased altitude, some evidence suggests that individuals with sickle cell trait have increased susceptibility to rhabdomyolysis, with the potential for renal failure and death.[80,81] Therefore, such individuals, like all athletes, should be carefully conditioned, acclimatized, and hydrated to reduce any possible risk when participating under extreme conditions.

Athletes with sickle cell disease require individual assessment for participation. Most often, these individuals are limited to low-intensity exercise because of increased sickling and crises due to hypoxemia and acidosis associated with more intense activities. Many patients self-restrict activities to avoid crises. However, if the status of the illness permits, all but high-exertion contact/collision sports may be played. Overheating, dehydration, and chilling must be avoided.

TESTICULAR DISORDERS

The incidence of scrotal injury requiring orchiectomy is extremely low in sports. Consensus is lacking on whether an athlete with a solitary functioning testicle should participate in contact/collision sports.[82] However, the athlete with a solitary testicle who wishes to participate in contact/collision sports must be informed that there is a risk of injury and loss of this testicle. Although wearing a protective cup may reduce the incidence of injury, it does not guarantee complete protection. Protective cups can be cumbersome and uncomfortable, and some athletes prefer not to wear them. However, with a thorough explanation of the potential benefits and availability of more comfortable cups, many athletes will choose to wear the protection and decrease their risk of injury.

If an athlete has an undescended testicle that has not been thoroughly evaluated, the examining physician should refer him for evaluation and inform him of the increased risk of testicular cancer. Clearance determination for an athlete who has an undescended testicle is similar to that for an athlete with a single testicle.

MEDICO*legal* CONSIDERATIONS

RIGHT TO PARTICIPATE

Three important medicolegal issues regarding the PPE have been receiving increasing scrutiny. The primary issue involves liability and assumption of risk when the athlete seeks to participate despite restrictions placed during the PPE. When an athlete has a condition for which the examining physician restricts participation in the desired sport, it is not uncommon for that athlete to seek another opinion or legal counsel to allow participation. Under such federal enactments as the Rehabilitation Act of 1973 and the Americans With Disabilities Act of 1990, the athlete may indeed have the legal right to participate against medical advice.[83]

Ideally, the physician who advises restricted participation should consult physicians with expertise in the medical condition in question to assist in determining the risk to the athlete of participating in the desired sport. Subsequently, it is imperative that the consulting physician(s) and the examining physician fully inform the athlete of any inherent risks of participation. This will allow the athlete to make an informed decision regarding participation. Such discussions should be well documented.

If the athlete chooses to participate despite contrary medical recommendations, some experts suggest that the athlete and his or her parent(s) or guardian(s) sign an exculpatory waiver or risk release to clearly indicate that they are fully informed of the inherent risk of participation against medical advice and that they assume this risk. An exculpatory waiver or risk release is a form of written contract between the athlete and his or her parent(s) or guardian(s), the physician, and the school or activity sponsor. In it, the athlete promises not to sue the physician or sponsor and releases the physician and sponsor from liability.[84] However, validity of these waivers may vary from state to state, and some experts question whether exculpatory waivers will adequately protect physicians from lawsuits.[85] Some institutions do not use exculpatory waivers, instead relying on the recommendations of medical personnel to determine clearance for participation. If the athlete is under the age of majority, his or her parent(s) or guardian(s) must sign the waiver; the physician must be aware of the age of majority in his or her state. Legal counsel is recommended on a case-by-case basis.

SEXUAL HARASSMENT CLAIMS

A second medicolegal issue has surfaced recently regarding professional conduct during the PPE. Occasionally, PPEs have led to allegations of provider sexual improprieties.[86] The mass station-based examination format may present the greatest risk of such claims, given the typical unfamiliarity of the patient-athlete with the examiner. Furthermore, athletes may not expect to have a thorough examination. Obviously, common sense should prevail. The physician should inform the athlete of the extent of the physical examination prior to performing it; provide an appropriate setting, possibly including "chaperones"; and use discretion with comments or actions that may be misconstrued. Furthermore, consistency in patient attire during the examination (eg, males in shorts with shirt removed, females in shorts and tank tops) and in the examination routine (eg, deferring female breast and genital examinations) will decrease the risk of an athlete's comparing his or her examination with those of other athletes and questioning why it might have been different.

GOOD SAMARITAN STATUTES

A third medicolegal consideration is the liability of those involved in performing PPEs on a volunteer basis. Until recently, Good Samaritan statutes did not release physicians from liability when providing PPEs free of charge. However, some states have taken measures to protect volunteer examiners and providers to athletic programs under Good Samaritan statutes.[87] It is important for physicians to know their state's statutes regarding PPEs and, if they wish to be protected by a Good Samaritan statute, be aware that they cannot accept any form of remuneration for their services.

CONCLUSION

Through genuine interest, thorough evaluation, and knowledgeable counseling, health care professionals can use the PPE as an opportunity to enhance the safety of sports participation. The PPE can also provide a "teachable moment" to discuss proper conditioning techniques, injury prevention, and lifestyle issues. This physician-athlete interaction may serve as the foundation for a trusting relationship, and for maximizing the athlete's long-term health.

REFERENCES

1. Linder CW, DuRant RH, Seklecki RM, et al: Preparticipation health screening of young athletes: results of 1268 examinations. Am J Sports Med 1981;9(3):187-193
2. Goldberg B, Saraniti A, Witman P, et al: Pre-participation sports assessment: an objective evaluation. Pediatrics 1980;66(5):736-745
3. Thompson TR, Andrish JT, Bergfeld JA: A prospective study of preparticipation sports examinations of 2670 young athletes: method and results. Cleve Clin Q 1982;49(4):225-233
4. Tennant FS Jr, Sorenson K, Day CM: Benefits of preparticipation sports examinations. J Fam Pract 1981;13(2):287-288
5. Magnes SA, Henderson JM, Hunter SC: What conditions limit sports participation? experience with 10,540 athletes. Phys Sportsmed 1992;20(5):143-160
6. McKeag DB: Preseason physical examination for the prevention of sports injuries. Sports Med 1985;2(6):413-431
7. Lombardo JA: Pre-participation physical evaluation. Prim Care 1984;11(1):3-21
8. Shaffer TE: The health examination for participation in sports. Pediatr Ann 1978;7(10):666-675
9. Risser WL, Hoffman HM, Bellah GG Jr: Frequency of preparticipation sports examinations in secondary school athletes: are the University Interscholastic League guidelines appropriate? Tex Med 1985;81(7):35-39
10. Kibler WB, Chandler TJ, Uhl T, et al: A musculoskeletal approach to the preparticipation physical examination: preventing injury and improving performance. Am J Sports Med 1989;17(4):525-531
11. Kibler WB, Chandler TJ: Sport specific screening and testing, in Renstrom P (ed): IOC Medical Commission, International Federation of Sports Medicine: Sports Injuries: Basic Principles of Prevention and Care. Oxford, Boston, Blackwell Scientific Pubs, 1993
12. Johnson MD, Kibler WB, Smith D, et al: Keys to successful preparticipation exams. Phys Sportsmed 1993;21(9):108-123
13. Lombardo JA, Robinson JB, Smith DM, et al: Preparticipation Physical Evaluation, ed 1. Kansas City, MO, American Academy of Family Physicians, American Academy of Pediatrics, American Medical Society for Sports Medicine, American Orthopaedic Society for Sports Medicine, American Osteopathic Academy of Sports Medicine, 1992
14. Committee on Sports Medicine: Sports Medicine: Health Care for Young Athletes. Evanston, IL, American Academy of Pediatrics, 1983
15. Dodge WF, West EF, Smith EH, et al: Proteinuria and hematuria in schoolchildren: epidemiology and early natural history. J Pediatr 1976;88(2):327-347
16. Peggs JF, Reinhardt RW, O'Brien JM: Proteinuria in adolescent sports physical examinations. J Fam Pract 1986;22(1):80-81
17. Taylor WC III, Lombardo JA: Preparticipation screening of college athletes: value of the complete blood cell count. Phys Sportsmed 1990;18(6):106-118
18. Vehaskari VM, Rapola J: Isolated proteinuria: analysis of a school-age population. J Pediatrics 1982;101(5):661-668
19. Ades PA: Preventing sudden death: cardiovascular screening of young athletes. Phys Sportsmed 1992;20(9):75-89
20. Epstein SE, Maron BJ: Sudden death and the competitive athlete: perspectives on preparticipation screening studies. J Am Coll Cardiol 1986;7(1):220-30
21. Feinstein RA, Colvin E, Oh MK: Echocardiographic screening as part of a preparticipation examination. Clin J Sport Med 1993;3(3):149-152
22. Lewis JF, Maron BJ, Diggs JA, et al: Preparticipation echocardiographic screening for cardiovascular disease in a large, predominantly black population of collegiate athletes. Am J Cardiol 1989;64(16):1029-1033
23. Maron BJ, Bodison SA, Wesley YE, et al: Results of screening a large group of intercollegiate competitive athletes for cardiovascular disease. J Am Coll Cardiol 1987;10(6):1214-1221
24. Rupp NT, Brudno DS, Guill MF: The value of screening for risk of exercise-induced asthma in high school athletes. Ann Allergy 1993;70(4):339-342
25. Rupp NT, Guill MF, Brudno DS: Unrecognized exercise-induced bronchospasm in adolescent athletes. Am J Dis Child 1992;146(8):941-944
26. Weidenbener EJ, Krauss MD, Waller BF, et al: Incorporation of screening echocardiography in the preparticipation exam. Clin J Sport Med 1995;5(2):86-89
27. Rice SG, Bierman CW, Shapiro GG, et al: Identification of exercise-induced asthma among intercollegiate athletes. Ann Allergy 1985;55(6):790-793
28. Shield S, Wang-Dohlman A: Incidence of exercise-induced bronchospasm in high school football players [abstract]. J Allergy Clin Immunol 1991;87(1 pt 2, suppl):166
29. Voy RO: The US Olympic Committee experience with exercise-induced bronchospasm 1984. Med Sci Sports Exerc 1986;18(3):328-330
30. Feinstein RA, La Russa J, Wang-Dohlman A, et al: Screening adolescent athletes for exercise-induced asthma. Clin J Sport Med 1996;6(2):119-123
31. Mitten MJ: HIV-positive athletes: when medicine meets the law. Phys Sportsmed 1994;22(10):63-68
32. American Medical Society for Sports Medicine (AMSSM) and American Academy of Sports Medicine (AASM) [American Orthopedic Society for Sports Medicine (AOSSM)]: Human immunodeficiency virus and other blood-borne pathogens in sports. Clin J Sport Med 1995;5(3):199-204
33. Rich BS: Sudden death screening. Med Clin North Am 1994;78(2):267-288
34. Van Camp SP: Sudden death in athletes, in Grana WA, Lombardo JA (eds): Advances in Sports Medicine and Fitness. Chicago, Year Book Medical Publishers, 1988, pp 121-142
35. Sallis RE, Jones K, Knopp W: Burners: offensive strategy for an under-reported injury. Phys Sportsmed 1992;20(11):47-55
36. American Academy of Pediatrics, American Academy of Ophthalmology: Protective Eyewear for Young Athletes. Pediatrics 1996;98(2):311-313
37. Tanner SM: Preparticipation examination targeted for the female athlete. Clin Sports Med 1994;13(2):337-353
38. Squire DL: Eating disorders, in Mellion MB (ed): Sports Medicine Secrets. Philadelphia, Hanley and Belfus, Inc; St Louis, Mosby, 1993, pp 136-141

39. Kiser C, Shank M, Kraemer W, et al: Effects of chewing tobacco on heart rate and blood pressure during exercise. J Sports Med Phys Fitness 1986;26:384-386
40. Edwards SE, Glover ED, Schroeder KL: The effects of smokeless tobacco on heart rate and neuromuscular reactivity in athletes and nonathletes. Phys Sportsmed 1987;15(7):141-147
41. Ferenchick GS, Adelman S: Myocardial infarction associated with anabolic steroid use in a previously healthy 37-year-old weight lifter. Am Heart J 1992;124(2):507-508
42. Hall B: The recommended childhood immunization schedule of the United States. Committee on Infectious Diseases, American Academy of Pediatrics, and Centers for Disease Control. Pediatrics 1995;95(1):135-137
43. American Academy of Pediatrics: Active and Passive Immunization, Section 1, in Peter O (ed): 1994 Red Book: Report of the Committee on Infectious Diseases, ed 23. Elk Grove Village, IL, American Academy of Pediatrics, 1994
44. Centers for Disease Control: Recommended childhood immunization schedule: United States, January-June 1996. MMWR Morb Mortal Wkly Rep 1996;44(51&52):940-943
45. American Heart Association: Cardiovascular Preparticipation Screening of Competitive Athletes. Circulation 1996;94(4):850-856
46. 26th Bethesda Conference: Recommendations for determining eligibility for competition in athletes with cardiovascular abnormalities. January 6-7, 1994. Med Sci Sports Exerc 1994;26(10 suppl):S223-283 [published erratum appears in Med Sci Sports Exerc 1994;26(12): following table of contents]; also in J Am Coll Cardiol 1994;24(4):845-899
47. Caine DJ, Broekhoff J: Maturity assessment: a viable preventive measure against physical and psychological insult to the young athlete? Phys Sportsmed 1987;15(3):67-80
48. Linder CW, et al: Preparticipation health screening of young athletes: results of 1,268 examinations. Am J Sports Med 1981;9(3):187-193
49. Gomez JE, Landry GL, Bernhardt DT: Critical evaluation of the 2-minute orthopedic screening examination. Am J Dis Child 1993;147(10):1109-1113
50. Smith DM: Preparticipation physical evaluations: development of uniform guidelines. Sports Med 1994;18(5):293-300
51. Stevens MB, Smith GN: The preparticipation sports assessment. Fam Pract Recert 1986;8(3):68-88
52. American Academy of Pediatrics Committee on Sports Medicine and Fitness: Medical conditions affecting sports participation. Pediatrics 1994;94(5):757-760
53. Mitchell JH, Haskell WL, Raven PB: Classification of sports, in 26th Bethesda Conference: Recommendations for determining eligibility for competition in athletes with cardiovascular abnormalities. Med Sci Sports Exerc 1994;26(10 suppl):S242-S245
54. Brown LS, Drotman P: What is the risk of HIV infection in athletic competition [abstract]. Presented at the Ninth International Conference on AIDS, Berlin, June 6-11, 1993
55. Goldsmith MF: When sports and HIV share the bill, smart money goes on common sense [news]. JAMA 1992;267(10):1311-1314
56. Guidelines for prevention of transmission of human immunodeficiency virus and hepatitis B virus to health-care and public-safety workers. MMWR Morb Mortal Wkly Rep 1989;38(suppl 6):1-37 [published erratum appears in MMWR Morb Mortal Wkly Rep 1989;38(43):746]
57. Ho DD, Moudgil T, Alam M: Quantitation of human immunodeficiency virus type 1 in the blood of infected persons. N Engl J Med 1989;321(24):1621-1625
58. Kashiwagi S, Hayashi J, Ikematsu H, et al: An outbreak of hepatitis B in members of a high school sumo wrestling club. JAMA 1982;248(2):213-214
59. Dolan PJ, Skibba RM, Hagan RC, et al: Hepatitis C: prevention and treatment. Am Fam Physician 1991;43(4):1347-1350, 1355-1360
60. Calabrese LH, LaPerriere A: Human immunodeficiency virus infection, exercise and athletics. Sports Med 1993;15(1):6-13
61. Maron BJ, Isner JM, McKenna WJ: Task Force 3: Hypertrophic cardiomyopathy, myocarditis and other myopericardial diseases and mitral valve prolapse, in 26th Bethesda Conference: Recommendations for determining eligibility for competition in athletes with cardiovascular abnormalities. Med Sci Sports Exerc 1994;26(10 suppl):S261-S267
62. Garner DM, Rosen LW: Eating disorders among athletes: research and recommendation. J App Sport Sci Res 1991;2(5):100-107
63. Vinger PF: Eye injuries, in Vinger PF, Hoerner EF (eds): Sports Injuries: The Unthwarted Epidemic, ed 2. Littleton, MA, PSG Pub Co, 1986, pp 146-147
64. Cantu RC: Guidelines for return to contact sports after a cerebral concussion. Phys Sportsmed 1986;14(10):75-83
65. Kelley JP, Nichols JS, Filley CM, et al: Concussion in sports: guidelines for the prevention of catastrophic outcome. JAMA 1991;266(20): 2867-2869
66. Sports Medicine Digest. Multiple concussion guidelines provoke controversy. Office of CME, UCLA School of Medicine, 1995;17(9):1-2
67. Sports Medicine Digest. Tough call: when is it safe to return to play after con-cussion? Office of CME, UCLA School of Medicine, 1995; 17(9):1,3,5-6
68. McCrory P, Maddocks D, Dicker G: Multiple concussive brain injury: lack of evidence for cumulative damage in a pilot study [abstract]. Med Sci Sports Exerc 1995:27(suppl to No. 5):S168
69. Sports Medicine Digest: Can repeated mild concussions cause long-term damage to the brain? 1995;17(9):6
70. Genarelli TA: Cerebral concussion and diffuse brain injuries, in Torg JS (ed): Athletic Injuries to the Head, Neck, and Face, ed 2. St Louis, Mosby Year Book, 1991, pp 170-182
71. Nelson WE, Jane JA, Gieck JH: Minor head injury in sports: a new system of classification and management. Phys Sportsmed 1984;12(3):103-107
72. Colorado Medical Society: Guidelines for the management of concussion in sports (revised). Denver, Colorado Medical Society, 1991
73. Mittenburg W, Burton DB: A survey of treatments for post-concussion syndrome. Brain Injury 1994;8(5):429-437
74. Saunders RL, Harbaugh RE: The second impact in catastrophic contact-sports head trauma. JAMA 1984;252(4):538-539
75. Cantu RC, Voy R: Second impact syndrome: a risk in any contact sport. Phys Sportsmed 1995;23(6):27-34
76. Torg JS: Management guidelines for athletic injuries to the cervical spine. Clin Sports Med 1987;6(1):53-60
77. Torg JS, Pavlov H, Genuario SE, et al: Neurapraxia of the cervical spinal cord with transient quadriplegia. J Bone Joint Surg (Am) 1986;68(9): 1354-1370
78. Torg JS, Glasgow SG: Criteria for return to contact activities following cervical spine injury. Clin J Sport Med 1991;1(1):12-26
79. Eichner ER: Sickle cell trait, exercise, and altitude. Phys Sportsmed 1986;14(11):144-157
80. Ramirez A, Hartley LH, Rhodes D, et al: Morphological features of red blood cells in subjects with sickle cell trait: changes during exercise. Arch Intern Med 1976;136(9):1064-1066
81. Eichner ER: Sickle cell trait, heroic exercise, and fatal collapse. Phys Sportsmed 1993;21(7):51-64
82. Dorsen PJ: Should athletes with one eye, kidney, or testicle play contact sports? Phys Sportsmed 1986;14(7):130-138
83. Gallup EM: Law and the Team Physician. Champaign, IL, Human Kinetics Books, 1995, pp 77, 80-81
84. *Ibid*, p 45
85. Herbert DL: Prospective releases: will their use protect sports medicine physicians from suit? Sports Med Stand Malpract Rep 1994;6(3):33, 35-36
86. Herbert DL: Professional considerations related to the conduct of preparticipation examinations. Sports Med Stand Malpract Rep 1994;6(4):49, 51-52
87. Gallup,[83] p 76-77

Preparticipation Physical Evaluation

HISTORY

DATE OF EXAM ______________

Name ______________ **Sex** ____ **Age** ____ **Date of birth** ______________

Grade ___ **School** ______________ **Sport(s)** ______________

Address ______________ **Phone** ______________

Personal physician ______________

In case of emergency, contact

Name ______________ **Relationship** ________ **Phone (H)** ______________ **(W)** ______________

Explain "Yes" answers below.
Circle questions you don't know the answers to.

	Yes	No
1. Have you had a medical illness or injury since your last check up or sports physical?	☐	☐
Do you have an ongoing or chronic illness?	☐	☐
2. Have you ever been hospitalized overnight?	☐	☐
Have you ever had surgery?	☐	☐
3. Are you currently taking any prescription or nonprescription (over-the-counter) medications or pills or using an inhaler?	☐	☐
Have you ever taken any supplements or vitamins to help you gain or lose weight or improve your performance?	☐	☐
4. Do you have any allergies (for example, to pollen, medicine, food, or stinging insects)?	☐	☐
Have you ever had a rash or hives develop during or after exercise?	☐	☐
5. Have you ever passed out during or after exercise?	☐	☐
Have you ever been dizzy during or after exercise?	☐	☐
Have you ever had chest pain during or after exercise?	☐	☐
Do you get tired more quickly than your friends do during exercise?	☐	☐
Have you ever had racing of your heart or skipped heartbeats?	☐	☐
Have you had high blood pressure or high cholesterol?	☐	☐
Have you ever been told you have a heart murmur?	☐	☐
Has any family member or relative died of heart problems or of sudden death before age 50?	☐	☐
Have you had a severe viral infection (for example, myocarditis or mononucleosis) within the last month?	☐	☐
Has a physician ever denied or restricted your participation in sports for any heart problems?	☐	☐
6. Do you have any current skin problems (for example, itching, rashes, acne, warts, fungus, or blisters)?	☐	☐
7. Have you ever had a head injury or concussion?	☐	☐
Have you ever been knocked out, become unconscious, or lost your memory?	☐	☐
Have you ever had a seizure?	☐	☐
Do you have frequent or severe headaches?	☐	☐
Have you ever had numbness or tingling in your arms, hands, legs, or feet?	☐	☐
Have you ever had a stinger, burner, or pinched nerve?	☐	☐
8. Have you ever become ill from exercising in the heat?	☐	☐
9. Do you cough, wheeze, or have trouble breathing during or after activity?	☐	☐
Do you have asthma?	☐	☐
Do you have seasonal allergies that require medical treatment?	☐	☐
10. Do you use any special protective or corrective equipment or devices that aren't usually used for your sport or position (for example, knee brace, special neck roll, foot orthotics, retainer on your teeth, hearing aid)?	☐	☐
11. Have you had any problems with your eyes or vision?	☐	☐
Do you wear glasses, contacts, or protective eyewear?	☐	☐
12. Have you ever had a sprain, strain, or swelling after injury?	☐	☐
Have you broken or fractured any bones or dislocated any joints?	☐	☐
Have you had any other problems with pain or swelling in muscles, tendons, bones, or joints?	☐	☐

If yes, check appropriate box and explain below.

☐ Head	☐ Elbow	☐ Hip
☐ Neck	☐ Forearm	☐ Thigh
☐ Back	☐ Wrist	☐ Knee
☐ Chest	☐ Hand	☐ Shin/calf
☐ Shoulder	☐ Finger	☐ Ankle
☐ Upper arm		☐ Foot

	Yes	No
13. Do you want to weigh more or less than you do now?	☐	☐
Do you lose weight regularly to meet weight requirements for your sport?	☐	☐
14. Do you feel stressed out?	☐	☐

15. Record the dates of your most recent immunizations (shots) for:

Tetanus ______________ Measles ______________

Hepatitis B ______________ Chickenpox ______________

FEMALES ONLY

16. When was your first menstrual period? ______________

When was your most recent menstrual period? ______________

How much time do you usually have from the start of one period to the start of another? ______________

How many periods have you had in the last year? ______________

What was the longest time between periods in the last year? _____

Explain "Yes" answers here: ______________

____

____

____

____

____

____

____

____

I hereby state that, to the best of my knowledge, my answers to the above questions are complete and correct.

Signature of athlete ______________ Signature of parent/guardian ______________ Date ______________

Preparticipation Physical Evaluation

PHYSICAL EXAMINATION

Name ______________________________ **Date of birth** ______________

Height ________ **Weight** ________ **% Body fat (optional)** ________ **Pulse** ______ **BP** ___/___ (___/___ , ___/___)

Vision R 20/ ____ **L 20/** ____ **Corrected: Y N** **Pupils: Equal** ____ **Unequal** ____

	NORMAL	ABNORMAL FINDINGS	INITIALS*
MEDICAL			
Appearance			
Eyes/Ears/Nose/Throat			
Lymph Nodes			
Heart			
Pulses			
Lungs			
Abdomen			
Genitalia (males only)			
Skin			
MUSCULOSKELETAL			
Neck			
Back			
Shoulder/arm			
Elbow/forearm			
Wrist/hand			
Hip/thigh			
Knee			
Leg/ankle			
Foot			

* Station-based examination only

CLEARANCE

❑ **Cleared**

❑ **Cleared after completing evaluation/rehabilitation for:** ______________________________

____

____

____

❑ **Not cleared for:** ______________ **Reason:** ______________

Recommendations: ______________________________

____

____

____

Name of physician (print/type) ______________________ **Date** __________

Address ______________________ **Phone** __________

Signature of physician ______________________, **MD or DO**

Preparticipation Physical Evaluation

CLEARANCE FORM

❑ **Cleared**

❑ **Cleared after completing evaluation/rehabilitation for:** ______________________

____

____

____

❑ **Not cleared for:** ______________________ **Reason:** ______________________

Recommendations: ______________________

____

____

____

Name of physician (print/type) ______________________ **Date** __________

Address ______________________ **Phone**__________

Signature of physician ______________________, **MD or DO**

Preparticipation Physical Evaluation

HISTORY

DATE OF EXAM ____________________

Name ______________________ **Sex** ______ **Age** ______ **Date of birth** ______________

Grade ____ **School** ______________ **Sport(s)** ______________________

Address ______________________________ **Phone** ______________

Personal physician ______________________________

In case of emergency, contact

Name ______________ **Relationship** __________ **Phone (H)** ______________ **(W)** ______________

Explain "Yes" answers below.
Circle questions you don't know the answers to.

	Yes	No
1. Have you had a medical illness or injury since your last check up or sports physical?	☐	☐
Do you have an ongoing or chronic illness?	☐	☐
2. Have you ever been hospitalized overnight?	☐	☐
Have you ever had surgery?	☐	☐
3. Are you currently taking any prescription or nonprescription (over-the-counter) medications or pills or using an inhaler?	☐	☐
Have you ever taken any supplements or vitamins to help you gain or lose weight or improve your performance?	☐	☐
4. Do you have any allergies (for example, to pollen, medicine, food, or stinging insects)?	☐	☐
Have you ever had a rash or hives develop during or after exercise?	☐	☐
5. Have you ever passed out during or after exercise?	☐	☐
Have you ever been dizzy during or after exercise?	☐	☐
Have you ever had chest pain during or after exercise?	☐	☐
Do you get tired more quickly than your friends do during exercise?	☐	☐
Have you ever had racing of your heart or skipped heartbeats?	☐	☐
Have you had high blood pressure or high cholesterol?	☐	☐
Have you ever been told you have a heart murmur?	☐	☐
Has any family member or relative died of heart problems or of sudden death before age 50?	☐	☐
Have you had a severe viral infection (for example, myocarditis or mononucleosis) within the last month?	☐	☐
Has a physician ever denied or restricted your participation in sports for any heart problems?	☐	☐
6. Do you have any current skin problems (for example, itching, rashes, acne, warts, fungus, or blisters)?	☐	☐
7. Have you ever had a head injury or concussion?	☐	☐
Have you ever been knocked out, become unconscious, or lost your memory?	☐	☐
Have you ever had a seizure?	☐	☐
Do you have frequent or severe headaches?	☐	☐
Have you ever had numbness or tingling in your arms, hands, legs, or feet?	☐	☐
Have you ever had a stinger, burner, or pinched nerve?	☐	☐
8. Have you ever become ill from exercising in the heat?	☐	☐
9. Do you cough, wheeze, or have trouble breathing during or after activity?	☐	☐
Do you have asthma?	☐	☐
Do you have seasonal allergies that require medical treatment?	☐	☐
10. Do you use any special protective or corrective equipment or devices that aren't usually used for your sport or position (for example, knee brace, special neck roll, foot orthotics, retainer on your teeth, hearing aid)?	☐	☐
11. Have you had any problems with your eyes or vision?	☐	☐
Do you wear glasses, contacts, or protective eyewear?	☐	☐
12. Have you ever had a sprain, strain, or swelling after injury?	☐	☐
Have you broken or fractured any bones or dislocated any joints?	☐	☐
Have you had any other problems with pain or swelling in muscles, tendons, bones, or joints?	☐	☐

If yes, check appropriate box and explain below.

☐ Head	☐ Elbow	☐ Hip
☐ Neck	☐ Forearm	☐ Thigh
☐ Back	☐ Wrist	☐ Knee
☐ Chest	☐ Hand	☐ Shin/calf
☐ Shoulder	☐ Finger	☐ Ankle
☐ Upper arm		☐ Foot

	Yes	No
13. Do you want to weigh more or less than you do now?	☐	☐
Do you lose weight regularly to meet weight requirements for your sport?	☐	☐
14. Do you feel stressed out?	☐	☐

15. Record the dates of your most recent immunizations (shots) for:

Tetanus ______________ Measles ______________

Hepatitis B ______________ Chickenpox ______________

FEMALES ONLY

16. When was your first menstrual period? ______________

When was your most recent menstrual period? ______________

How much time do you usually have from the start of one period to the start of another? ______________

How many periods have you had in the last year? ______________

What was the longest time between periods in the last year? ______

Explain "Yes" answers here: ______________________________

____

____

____

____

____

____

____

____

____

I hereby state that, to the best of my knowledge, my answers to the above questions are complete and correct.

Signature of athlete ______________ Signature of parent/guardian ______________ Date ______________

Preparticipation Physical Evaluation

PHYSICAL EXAMINATION

Name ______________________________ **Date of birth** ______________

Height ________ **Weight** ________ **% Body fat (optional)** ________ **Pulse** ______ **BP** ___/___ (___/___ , ___/___)

Vision R 20/ _____ **L 20/** _____ **Corrected: Y N** **Pupils: Equal** _____ **Unequal** _____

	NORMAL	ABNORMAL FINDINGS	INITIALS*
MEDICAL			
Appearance			
Eyes/Ears/Nose/Throat			
Lymph Nodes			
Heart			
Pulses			
Lungs			
Abdomen			
Genitalia (males only)			
Skin			
MUSCULOSKELETAL			
Neck			
Back			
Shoulder/arm			
Elbow/forearm			
Wrist/hand			
Hip/thigh			
Knee			
Leg/ankle			
Foot			

* Station-based examination only

CLEARANCE

❑ **Cleared**

❑ **Cleared after completing evaluation/rehabilitation for:** ______________________________

____

____

____

❑ **Not cleared for:** ______________ **Reason:** ______________

Recommendations: ______________________________

____

____

____

Name of physician (print/type) ______________________________ **Date** ______________

Address ______________________________ **Phone** ______________

Signature of physician ______________________________, **MD or DO**

Preparticipation Physical Evaluation

CLEARANCE FORM

❑ **Cleared**

❑ **Cleared after completing evaluation/rehabilitation for:** ______________________________

____

____

____

❑ **Not cleared for:** ____________________ **Reason:** ____________________

Recommendations: ______________________________

____

____

____

Name of physician (print/type) ______________________________ **Date** __________

Address ______________________________ **Phone**__________

Signature of physician ______________________________**, MD or DO**

Preparticipation Physical Evaluation

CLEARANCE FORM

❑ **Cleared**

❑ **Cleared after completing evaluation/rehabilitation for:** ______________________________

____

____

____

❑ **Not cleared for:** ____________________ **Reason:** ____________________

Recommendations: ______________________________

____

____

____

Name of physician (print/type) ______________________________ **Date** __________

Address ______________________________ **Phone**__________

Signature of physician ______________________________**, MD or DO**

© 1997 *American Academy of Family Physicians, American Academy of Pediatrics, American Medical Society for Sports Medicine, American Orthopaedic Society for Sports Medicine, and American Osteopathic Academy of Sports Medicine.*

ISBN 0-07-001627-5
90000>
9 780070 016279